547039 6/1

£45.60

GLENSIDE HOSPITAL

MEDICAL LIBRARY

GW01486371

Interface between Neurology and Psychiatry

Advances in Psychosomatic Medicine

Vol. 13

Series Editor
Thomas N. Wise, Falls Church, Va.

Editors
G. Fava, Bologna; *H. Freyberger,* Hannover;
F. Guggenheim, Dallas, Tex.; *O.W. Hill,* London;
Z.J. Lipowski, Toronto; *G. Lloyd,* Edinburgh;
J.C. Nemiah, Boston, Mass.; *A. Reading,* Tampa, Fla.;
P. Reich, Boston, Mass.

Consulting Editors
G.L. Engel, Rochester, N.Y.; *H. Weiner,* Bronx, N.Y.;
L. Levi, Stockholm

Editor Emeritus
Franz Reichsman, Brooklyn, N.Y.

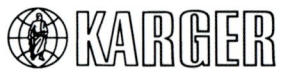

Basel · München · Paris · London · New York · New Delhi · Singapore · Tokyo · Sydney

Interface between Neurology and Psychiatry

Volume Editor
M.R. Trimble, London

11 figures and 12 tables, 1985

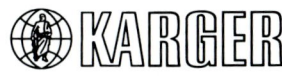

Basel · München · Paris · London · New York · New Delhi · Singapore · Tokyo · Sydney

Advances in Psychosomatic Medicine

National Library of Medicine, Cataloging in Publication
　　Interface between neurology and psychiatry/
　　volume editor, M.R. Trimble.
　　– Basel; New York: Karger, 1985 –
　　(Advances in psychosomatic medicine; vol. 13)
　　Includes index.
　　1. Nervous System Diseases – psychology 2. Psychophysiologic Disorders I. Trimble, Michel R. II. Series
　　W1 AD81 v. 13 [WM 90 I595]
　　ISBN 3–8055–4023–X

Drug Dosage
　　The authors and the publisher have exerted every effort to ensure that drug selection and dosage set forth in this text are in accord with current recommendations and practice at the time of publication. However, in view of ongoing research, changes in government regulations, and the constant flow of information relating to drug therapy and drug reactions, the reader is urged to check the package insert for each drug for any change in indications and dosage and for added warnings and precautions. This is particularly important when the recommended agent is a new and/or infrequently employed drug.

All rights reserved.
　　No part of this publication may be translated into other languages, reproduced or utilized in any form or by any means, electronic or mechanical, including photocopying, recording, microcopying, or by any information storage and retrieval system, without permission in writing from the publisher.
　　© Copyright 1985 by S. Karger AG, P.O. Box, CH–4009 Basel (Switzerland)
　　Printed in Switzerland by Boehm-Hutter AG, Reinach BL
　　ISBN 3–8055–4023–X

Contents

Introduction
   M.R. Trimble, London VII

1. Emotional Behaviour and the Limbic System
   J.A. Gray, London 1
2. The Social Environment and Neurological Disease
   I. Grant, La Jolla, Calif. 26
3. Head Injury, Neurosis and Accident Proneness
   A.C.P. Sims, Leeds 49
4. Emotional Aspects of Cerebrovascular Disease
   P. Storey, London 71
5. Psychosomatic Aspects of Multiple Sclerosis
   J.W. Paulley, Ipswich 85
6. Psychosomatic Aspects of Movement Disorders
   J.L. Cummings, Los Angeles, Calif. 111
7. Psychosomatic Aspects of Epilepsy
   M.R. Trimble, London 133
8. Behavioural Psychotherapy for Neurological Illness
   J. Cobb, London 151

Subject Index 185

Introduction

Although psychosomatic medicine is a relatively recently developed concept, psychosomatic principals in medicine have a long history [*Lipowski,* 1984]. Many physicians have noted and acknowledged the role of stress and trauma in the initiation or progression of various disease states, culminating with the development of clearly defined psychosomatic theories regarding these links in the earlier part of this century. The converse, namely the associations between somatic disease and psychological disturbance, has too been the concern of many, from observations that various secondary effects of disease impair brain function ('exogenous' reaction types) to the more subtle effects of chronic disease on the development of personality and the precipitation of psychopathology. Unfortunately, although the stated intention was often otherwise, many writers in these areas have persistently supported the inherent dualism, known as 'Cartesian dualism' which, instead of presenting psychosomatic concepts as unifying with regards to the mind/body problem, display clearly the pons asinorum which has been so destructive to this area.

The recent rise in interest in psychosomatics may be said to start in the 1930s with the writings of *Dunbar* [1935], and the inauguration of the *Journal of Psychosomatic Medicine* [*Lipowski,* 1984]. These beginnings were, however, confused with the abundant theorising of the psychoanalysts, and some of the conceptions with regards to psychosomatic mechanisms were entirely construed as one way traffic, for example in the propositions of *Groddeck* [1961] which linked all illness to symbolic mechanisms and conflict. *Alexander* [1950] invoking 'the ductless glands' and the 'vegatative nervous system' in the pathogenesis of disease acknowledged that 'the unity of the organism is clearly expressed in the functions of the central nervous system ... represented by the highest centres'. However, any more precise description of *which* parts of the brain were involved or how appeared lacking. However, earlier suggestions regarding the involvement of the central nervous system in psychosomatic illness had stemmed from the writings of *Cannon* and *Pavlov*. *Canon's* work on the role of the sympathetic nervous system in the motor expression of rage and fear, and the connections of the autonomic system to the gastrointestinal tract were discussed by *Dunbar* [1935], and provided an impetus to the well-known pioneering work of *Harold Wolff* [*Meyer*, 1959]. *Gantt's* work follows from *Pavlov* and the influence of conditioned reflexes on behaviour [*Meyer*, 1959], leading to a whole range of behaviour therapies which are in use today for the treatment of psychosomatic ailments (see *Cobb*, chapt. 8).

Discovery of the reticular activating system, a collection of neurones deep in the mid- and hind-brain structures led to further speculations of the role in CNS factors in psychosomatic relationships. However, the real breakthrough in providing a more tenable hypothesis of the role of the brain in psychosomatic mechanisms came with the writings of *Papez* [1937] and *MacLean* [1970]. *Papez* noted a distinction between the activities of the medial cortex, especially the hippocampus and cingulate cortex, which participate in hypothalamic activities, and the lateral neocortex mediating general sensory activity. The *Papez* circuit, comprising of the hippocampal formation, the mamillary bodies, the anterior thalamic nuclei and the gyrus cinguli was suggested as central in the elaboration of affective experience. *MacLean* [1970] formulated more convincingly the concept of the limbic *system,* comprising a collection of tracts and neurones of phylogenetically older cortex that played 'a basic role in integrating emotional expression'. Further, he postulated a mechanism for explanation of psychosomatic phenomena involving the limbic system and its connections to the hypothalamus. Anticipating the concept of alexithymia he wrote: 'in the psychosomatic patient it would almost seem there was little direct exchange between the visceral brain and the word brain and that emotional feelings built up in the hippocampal formation, instead of being relayed to the intellect for evaluation found immediate expression through autonomic centres ...' [*MacLean*, 1949].

Recent work has considerably expanded our knowledge of both the neuroanatomy and neurochemistry of this system and its role in behaviour and emotional expression. While the anatomical details of these brain structures can be found in other texts [*Trimble*, 1981; *Isaacson*, 1974] the full impact of this development in our understanding of brain function has not clearly reached the interstices of psychiatric and psychosomatic thought. Thus, for the first time, there is some identifiable neurological link mediating between those cortical areas that receive information regarding the environment and the situation of the individual and the neuronal systems that relay information regarding the self. The latter derive from internal receptors for sensory information from the body, projecting to diencephalic structures, especially providing information relating to elements of behaviour such as pain, hunger and sexual arousal, vital for survival. Indeed, if the concept of the limbic system and its relationship to emotion is acknowledged, then we have, from a neurological viewpoint, a much clearer hypothesis to work with when we speak of 'emotional disorders'. Thus, in the same way that now, some one hundred years after Broca, we accept that speech disorders somehow relate to disturbance of brain function in those areas of the central nervous system that mediate speech, the term 'emotional disorders' links immediately to the limbic system and its dysregulation. This in no way precludes the necessity to acknowledge that social and environmental factors are linked to such dysfunction, since it is clear that a vast amount of sensory information about our environment is channelled directly to limbic system structures via temporal cortical areas and the entorhinal cortex. Further, it does not exclude a reciprocal link between the limbic system and cortex, such that disturbances from the former may readily impair the reception of sensory information in the latter leading to distortions of evaluation and interpretation. Most neuroanatomically defined pathways between limbic system structures and neocortex, and indeed within the limbic system itself, admit two way traffic, emphasising the constant interplay, obvious to us all, between emotion and cognition.

In view of this importance of the limbic system for any neurological understanding of the emotions, this book, devoted as it is to a further exploration of the links between psychosomatic disorder and neurology, begins with a chapter by Prof. *Gray* on animal models of the limbic system, especially the septo-hippocampal links to anxiety and possibly some forms of depression. There is, however, another reason to start with the writings of Prof. *Gray*. It is clear that much interesting work is being undertaken in laboratory animals that has relevance for clinical problems, and a good example of this is the attempt to explore animal models of anxiety seeking the underlying contributions of neurochemistry, neurophysiology and neuroanatomy to the clinical problems we encounter. In this chapter, the central role of the limbic system in mediating anxiety is emphasised as well as some psychosomatic links suggested. The limbic system, with the hypothalamus, hence pituitary gland, as one of its major output pathways, influences not only a wide variety of autonomic phenomena but also neuroendocrine output. The possible associations between altered hormone output and stress has had a long tradition in psychosomatic medicine, but newer possibilities, including the interaction between hormones (expecially steroids and more recently peptides) and immune capacity must have relevance for an understanding of psychosomatic mechanisms and provide good grounds for further research.

Another important way to view the interaction between the central nervous system and morbidity, with psychosomatic overtones is through the interaction of personality, accident proneness and head injuries, discussed in the chapter by Prof. *Sims*. This follows a review of some of the ways that psychosocial events, especially life events, may be related to the precipitation or continuation of neurological diseases. Life events research, as Prof. *Grant* illustrates, is in its relative infancy, and yet there are clear hints and suggestions, especially with some neurological diseases that life events somehow relate to both morbidity and mortality.

The following four chapters emphasise some of the psychosomatic links that may be derived from the literature in selective neurological diseases. Dr. *Storey* covers the highly relevant field of cerebrovascular disease, Dr. *Paulley* that of multiple sclerosis, Dr. *Cummings* covers a range of motor disorders and the Editor's contribution is on epilepsy. Each of these authors has approached the topic in a different way. For example, Dr. *Paulley* not only reviews a fascinating literature in detail but also gives guidance for 'common sense psychotherapy', reviewing its use in the tragic condition of multiple sclerosis. The role of pre-morbid personality in the pathogenesis of this disorder is revived, emphasising a recent renewed interest in exploring links between personality and illness, which at the present time is flowering most successfully in the cardiological literature in relationship to myocardial disease and type A and B personalities. Dr. *Cummings* extends the concept of psychosomatic considerably, and in seeking neurological underpinnings includes subcortical links to basal ganglia structures. He provides us with both clinical and anatomical evidence to extend our understanding to include movement in association with emotion and cognition, (a 'moving experience' implies an emotional one in the English language, and the word 'jerk' is used both as a pejorative expression of a person's character and a clearly defined movement).

Finally, Dr. *Cobb* presents an overview, but with practical advice, on the management of some neurological conditions with behavioural methods. Such techniques seem often to provide relief for otherwise intractable problems, although as Dr. *Cobb* points out they require further controlled investigation and do not represent a panacea.

It is hoped that the interested reader will gain encouragement to seek further information regarding some of the links between psychosomatics and the central nervous system briefly discussed in this work. The Editor is grateful to all those who have contributed to this volume, and is aware that other topics could have been included (pain is an obvious example), but in the space available selection was important and an attempt has been made to emphasise some of the less well discussed areas of this growing interface.

References

Alexander, F.: Psychosomatic medicine (Norton, New York 1950).
Dunbar, H.: Emotions and bodily changes: a survey of literature on psychosomatic inter-relationships (1910–1933) (Columbia Press, New York 1935).
Groddeck, G.: The book of the it. (Vintage Books, New York 1961).
Isaacson, R.L.: The limbic system (Plenum Press, New York 1974).
Lipowsky, Z.J.: What does the word psychosomatic really mean? A historical and semantic enquiry. Psychosom. Med. *46:* 153–171 (1984).
MacLean, P.D.: Psychosomatic disease and the visceral brain. Psychosom. Med. *11:* 338–353 (1949).
MacLean, P.D.: The triune brain, emotion of scientific basis; in The Neurosciences Second Study Programme, pp. 336–349 (Rockefeller University Press, New York 1970).
Meyer, E.: The psychosomatic concept, use and abuse. J. chron. Dis. *9:* 298–314 (1959).
Papez, J.W.: A proposed mechanism of emotion. Archs Neurol. Psychiat. *38:* 725–743 (1937).
Trimple, M.R.: The limbic system; in Reynolds, Trimble, Epilepsy and psychiatry, pp. 216–226 (Churchill Livingstone, Edinburgh 1981).

M.R. Trimble, London 1984

Michael R. Trimble, MRCP, FRCPsych., Consultant Physician in Psychological Medicine, The National Hospitals, London WC1N 3BG (UK)

1. Emotional Behaviour and the Limbic System

J.A. Gray

Department of Psychology, Institute of Psychiatry, London, UK

Introduction

As the old slogan had it, 'no psychosis without neurosis'. The meaning of these words has now changed, so that a translation into contemporary English is needed: no mental illness without disturbance in brain function. This principle remains valid today, and its validity extends to the field of psychosomatic diseases: psyche affects soma by way of its material substrate, the brain (and soma, of course, affects psyche by the same route). One further act of translation is needed to bring this preamble up to date: by 'psyche' is meant the systems that control behaviour. There are therefore four terms in the interactions that concern us: the body (soma), behaviour, the systems that control behaviour (psyche), and the brain. An earlier fashionable contrast for the last two of these terms (psyche and brain) qualified them as the 'conceptual' and the 'real' nervous systems; a more recent one contrasts them as 'software' and 'hardware'.

The mental states that have most often been implicated in the genesis and maintenance of psychosomatic illness are the emotions. It would seem therefore that full understanding of psychosomatic illness will require a successful analysis of the brain mechanisms that mediate the emotions and of their input-output relations with the body. We are still a long way short of possessing such an analysis – so far short, indeed, that any attempt even to list the different emotions (assuming that they can eventually be differentiated one from the other) would be at the moment a highly speculative enterprise. In this chapter, therefore, I shall concentrate on those aspects of the emotions and emotional behaviour about which one can say something concrete. This strategy will narrow my scrutiny to anxiety, depression and the development of tolerance for stress; and even in this foreshortened list, as we shall see, there is doubt as to whether one can distinguish the brain mechanisms that underlie anxiety and depression respectively.

Anxiety is probably the emotion that has most often been related clinically to psychosomatic symptoms; it is also, I believe, the emotion whose neurology is at present most fully understood. It is therefore the most natural place at which to start.

The Neurology of Anxiety

An obvious problem in studying the neural basis of any mental state is that one cannot do experiments with the only organisms – people – that can attempt to describe their mental states (though, to be sure, such descriptions are in any case notoriously fallible). We can glean what information we can from the random insults to the brain that accident and disease cause our fellows; but, for systematic research, we have no alternative but to make use of animals. However, we then face the equally difficult problem of determining what mental states the subjects of our experiments experience. Stated this way the problem is not merely difficult, it is apparently intractable. But it can be reduced to manageable proportions by making use of the translation rules we have just established. A mental state is a state of the systems that control behaviour. Furthermore, such a state is inferred from observations of behaviour and used to account for and predict behaviour – a formulation that is as true when applied to people as when applied to rats, cats or monkeys. It is thus no harder (and, given the relatively greater simplicity of their behaviour, may even be easier) to do this for animals than for people. We can at the very least subject our inferences about the emotional states of, say, a laboratory rat to systematic and rigorous experimental test – something rarely if ever possible with human beings in or out of the laboratory. So the problem lies, not in the ascription of mental states to animals, but in determining the equivalence of the states so ascribed to those experienced by people. In short, the question that must first concern us here is: Is it possible to ascribe to experimental animals a state sufficiently similar to the human state of anxiety to allow one to study the neurology of anxiety in animals?

I have posed and answered this question at some length elsewhere [*Gray,* 1982a, b]. The solution to our problem turns on the use as an experimental tool of the anti-anxiety drugs (including principally the benzo-

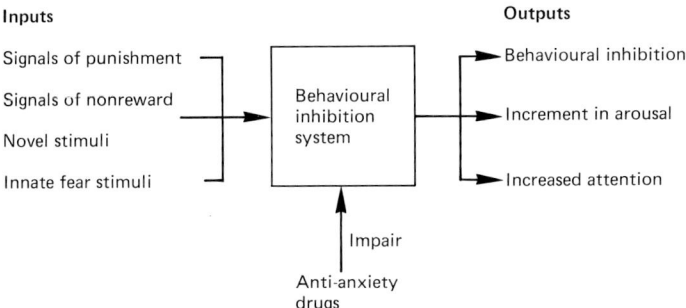

Fig. 1. The behavioral inhibition system. This responds to any of its adequate inputs with all of its outputs, and comprises the hypothetical substrate on which the anti-anxiety drugs act to reduce anxiety.

diazepines, the barbiturates and alcohol) [*Gray*, 1977]. These drugs appear to be effective in the acute control of anxiety in man [*Rickels*, 1978]. Can we then use them to ask (by studying their mode of action in the brain) what neural mechanisms mediate anxiety? The answer to this question is a conditional 'yes' – but the condition is a hard one to meet: we must first show that the behavioural effects of the anti-anxiety drugs in animals are consistent with the hypothesis that animals possess a mental state similar to human anxiety and that this state is reduced by the action of the drugs. (The same condition, mutatis mutandis, applies to the use of all psychotropic agents as probes of animal mental states, but it is one that is normally more honoured in the breach than in the observance.)

In an attempt to see whether this condition can be met, I have reviewed some 400 experiments in which one or other of the anti-anxiety drugs have been administered to species ranging from goldfish to chimpanzees [*Gray*, 1977]. The results of the very diverse procedures that have been used in these experiments yield to a satisfyingly simple set of generalisations (summarised in fig. 1). One may account for the great majority of the experimental findings by the following rules. First, three kinds of stimuli are functionally equivalent in the types of behavioural change they elicit; these are stimuli associated with pain or punishment, stimuli associated with nonreward (i.e. the non-occurrence of anticipated reward) or failure, and novel stimuli (left-hand side of fig. 1); other kinds of stimuli (including pain and nonreward as such) do not elicit same types of behavioural change. Second, the types of behavioural change elicited by these stimuli consist in inhibition of ongoing behaviour, increased level of arousal (so that the next initiated behavioural act is performed harder or faster than usual), and increased attention to the environment and especially novel elements in the environment (right-hand side of fig. 1). Third, all these types of behavioural change in response to any of the appropriate stimuli are reduced by administration of any of the anti-anxiety drugs.

One can interpret these findings by supposing (1) that the brain contains a special-purpose system (the behavioural inhibition system in fig. 1) whose behavioural outputs (listed to the right of fig. 1) occur in response to any of the inputs listed to the left, and (2) that activity in the behavioural inhibition system is counteracted by the anti-anxiety drugs. We next go one step further and postulate (3) that activity in the behavioural inhibition system constitutes the mental state of anxiety. We can now state that anxiety is (in every-day language) a state produced by the threat of pain, punishment, nonreward or failure, or by an encounter with a novel or uncertain environment; and that, in a state of anxiety, one 'stops, looks and listens' and prepares for hard and rapid action. This, I think, would be recognised by the proverbial man on the Clapham omnibus as a plausible account of human anxiety, yet it is entirely based upon experiments with animals. It is this fact which gives me courage to suppose that animals possess a state of anxiety that is closely similar to the human state bearing that name.

If this conclusion is accepted, several others flow from it. First, note that the generalisations summarised in figure 1 appear to apply equally well to all the species tested, from goldfish to chimpanzees (although the great bulk of the data have come from experiments with rodents). This implies that anxiety is phylogenetically old and depends neither on the great growth of the neocortex in man nor on the recognition of one's own mortality nor on the stresses of modern life nor yet on the Oedipus complex. This conclusion is backed up by biochemical evidence, which demonstrates that the high-affinity specific benzodiazepine receptor recently shown to be located on neuronal membranes [*Möhler and Okada,* 1977; *Braestrup and Squires,* 1977] is present in the same form in higher bony fish and in mammals including man [*Nielsen* et al., 1978]. Phylogenetic longevity in turn implies that anxiety is functionally useful – it is not there to bring some of us into hospital but because, in our evolutionary past, it has helped all of us to survive. The same line of argument leads to a further important conclusion: we may seek in the brains of animals for a phylogenetically stable neural substrate of anxiety and have some hope of finding it.

These considerations guide our search towards structures older than that late-flowering plant (phylogenetically speaking), the neocortex. Other sign-posts point in the same direction: a wealth of evidence from experiments in which the brain has been lesioned in diverse manners, or stimulated electrically or chemically, implicates as the heartland of emotional experience the complex of interlinked structures that make up the limbic system [*Isaacson*, 1974] perhaps together with the hypothalamus [*Panksepp*, 1982]. It is here, therefore, that we should start searching for the neural substrate of anxiety.

There are two rather different ways of going about this search. The first and obvious way is to ask directly of the anti-anxiety drugs what they do in the brain – to membranes, synapses, receptors, transmitters and the like. But this direct approach runs into difficulties. Like all drugs, anti-anxiety drugs have more than one kind of effect: besides reducing anxiety, they are (among other things) muscle relaxants, sedatives and anti-convulsants. Discovery, therefore, that anti-anxiety drugs have such-and-such an effect on, say, a receptor fails to tell us that this effect is related to anxiety reduction, because it could equally well underlie some other 'side effect' (from our point of view) of the drug. While this problem is general in the analysis of drug action, it is particularly acute in regard to the anti-anxiety drugs, since their best-documented biochemical effect (clear for both benzodiazepines and barbiturates and possibly involved also in the action of alcohol) is to enhance the synaptic efficacy of the inhibitory neurotransmitter, γ-aminobutyric acid (GABA) [*Costa*, 1983]. The benzodiazepines do this by way of their specific receptor, which is closely coupled to GABA receptors [*Bowery*, 1984], the barbiturates perhaps by way of yet another receptor forming part of the same supramolecular complex [*Olsen*, 1981]. But GABA (and benzodiazepine) receptors are distributed throughout the central nervous system, including the spinal cord, so this fact about the neurochemical actions of anti-anxiety drugs barely narrows at all the range of possible sites at which the brain might mediate anxiety. What we have instead is an excellent means of anti-convulsant action – the deepening of a general inhibitory blanket on the brain.

In the absence of more specific indications of the neural basis of anxiety from the direct approach, we must supplement our search by an indirect approach to the problem. This is the approach favoured by psychologists, to whom it is natural to ask (fig. 1): 'What can I do to the brain which will mimic the actions of the anti-anxiety drugs in behavioural tests that are sensitive to the functions of the behavioural inhibition system?'

Or: 'What can I do to the brain which will produce effects in such tests that are diametrically opposed to those of the anti-anxiety drugs?' Answers to these questions should pin-point those regions of the brain that are crucial to anti-anxiety behavioural action (though, to be sure, we shall also need to demonstrate how the known neurochemical actions of the drugs can give rise to altered functioning in these regions of the brain).

These too are questions that I have considered extensively elsewhere [*Gray*, 1982a, b]. Before I outline the conclusions I reached, a word of caution is in order. We should not expect to uncover any simple one-to-one mapping between structures in the brain and concepts in our psychology. If we are correct in delineating a separate psychological state, e.g. that of anxiety, it follows that there are structures in the brain which mediate that state; but it does not follow either that these structures will themselves be neatly separable from other brain structures nor that they discharge only one set of functions corresponding to only one psychological state. There is almost bound to be, in other words, only partial overlap between psychological concepts and anatomical boundaries: a given psychological function will require many structures for its discharge, and the structures may themselves vary in relation to the exact manner in which the function is discharged; and a given structure will play a role in the discharge of many different functions. These important caveats must not be lost from sight in the dogmatic summary of conclusions that follows.

Chief among these conclusions is that a central role in the neuropsychology of anxiety is played by the septo-hippocampal system [*Elliot and Whelan,* 1978]. The major (but not the only) item of evidence upon which this conclusion rests is the remarkable similarity that exists between the behavioural syndrome observed after administration of the anti-anxiety drugs [*Gray,* 1977], on the one hand, and lesions to the septal area or hippocampal formation [*Gray and McNaughton,* 1983] on the other. The extent of this similarity is so great that it is difficult to believe that the anti-anxiety drugs do not include an impairment in the functioning of the septo-hippocampal system as one of their major paths of action. This conclusion is in no way inconsistent with the evidence that the mode of action of these substances includes an enhancement of GABAergic inhibition. There are many routes by which such enhanced inhibition might give rise to reduced activity in the septo-hippocampal system, including increased efficacy of GABA within the hippocampal formation or septal area themselves. One particular route, however, appears to be especially important (though not necessarily to the exclusion of others). Ascending monoaminergic inputs

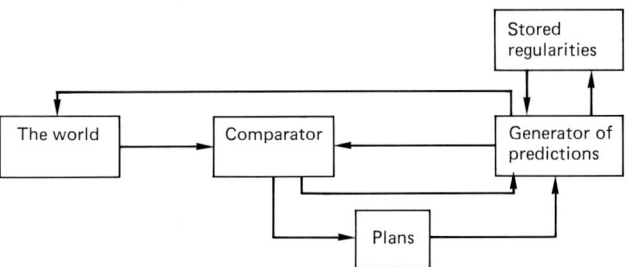

Fig. 2. The kinds of information processing required for the successful functioning of the hypothetical comparator (see text for further information).

(both noradrenergic and serotonergic) to the septo-hippocampal system appear to increase the efficiency with which this system processes afferents from the neocortex (via the entorhinal area) [*Segal*, 1977]. These inputs are expecially active under conditions of stress, and this stress-induced increment in their activity is reversed by the anti-anxiety drugs [*Lidbrink* et al., 1972]. Blockade of the noradrenergic input to the septo-hippocampal system by these drugs could be secondary to enhanced GABAergic inhibition at the cell bodies in the locus coeruleus (in the brain stem) or at terminals within the septal area or hippocampus [*Gray* et al., 1984]; similarly, blockade of the serotonergic input could be secondary to enhanced GABAergic inhibition at the cell bodies in the median raphe nucleus or at septo-hippocampal terminals.

Knowledge of the brain regions that mediate a psychological state is an important step forward. But it is an incomplete step unless one can supplement this information with an understanding of the particular functions discharged by these brain regions and the manner in which they contribute to the psychological state in question. We do not yet possess such an understanding for anxiety (or for any emotion). However, speculation is possible, and I have indulged in it elsewhere [*Gray*, 1982a, b]. The central tenet of this speculation is that the septo-hippocampal system, together with its neocortical input (from the entorhinal area) and its connections to *Papez'* [1937] circuit (subicular area, mammillary bodies, anteromedial thalamus and cingulate cortex), discharges the function of a comparator (see fig. 2), matching (1) sensory inputs describing the current state of the organism's world to (2) predictions (generated within the same system) as to what those inputs should be. When sensory inputs and predicted inputs

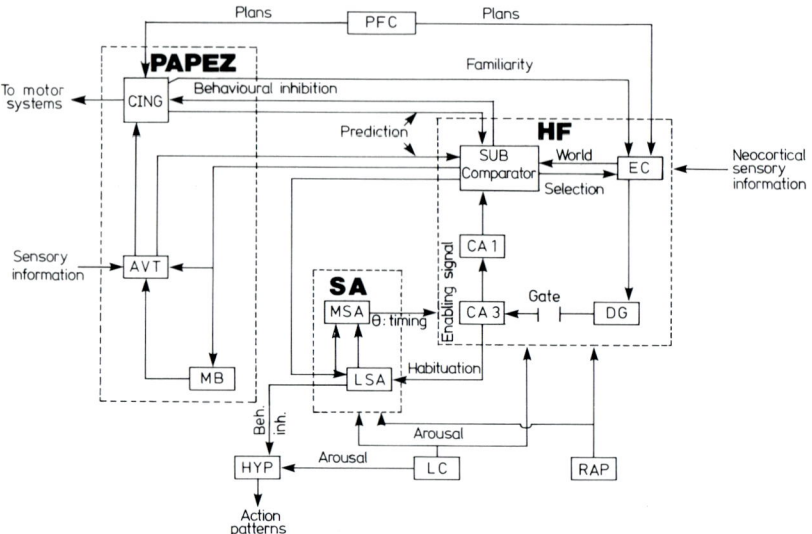

Fig. 3. A summary of the theory developed in *Gray* [1982a, b]. The three major building blocks are shown in heavy print: HF, the hippocampal formation, made up of the entorhinal cortex, EC, the dentate gyrus, DG, CA_3, CA_1, and the subicular area, SUB; SA, the septal area, containing the medial and lateral septal areas, MSA and LSA; and the Papez circuit, which receives projections from and returns them to the subicular area via the mammillary bodies, MB, anteroventral thalamus, AVT, and cingulate cortex, CING. Other structures shown are the hypothalamus, HYP, the locus coeruleus, LC, the raphe nuclei, RAP, and the prefrontal cortex, PFC. Arrows show direction of projection; the projection from SUB to LSA lacks anatomical confirmation. Words in lower case show postulated functions (for further explanation, *see Gray* [1982a, b].

can be successfully matched, this system confines itself to a monitoring function and behaviour is controlled by other regions of the brain. When a 'mismatch' occurs (something happens that is not predicted, something that is predicted fails to happen, or something that is predicted is aversive) then the septo-hippocampal system takes control of behaviour and operates the outputs of the behavioural inhibition system (fig. 1). It would take us too far afield to go into the details of this model of septo-hippocampal function here; its flavour is to some extent captured in figure 3.

Within the framework of this model, anxiety can be conceptualised in two ways. One way is to treat the degree of anxiety as proportional to the number of items that the comparator selects for processing (that is, for prediction and matching to the world). Viewed in this manner, a high level of anxiety corresponds quite well to the kinds of symptoms displayed by patients with the obsessive-compulsive syndrome: an over-zealous checking of the environment and one's own behaviour, and vigilance for the dangers that may be attendant on both. The second way treats anxiety as proportional to the ease with which the comparator declares 'mismatch' and operates the outputs of the behavioural inhibition system. Viewed like this, anxiety corresponds to the kind of symptom displayed by patients with wide-ranging phobias (e.g. agoraphobia). These two ways of looking at anxiety are not mutually exclusive – rather the reverse, since the more items that are monitored the greater is the likelihood (other things being equal) that some discrepancy will be noticed. The frequent co-existence, clinically, of obsessional and phobic symptoms, therefore, is to be expected, given the model. The monoaminergic (especially the noradrenergic) inputs to the septo-hippocampal system (whose activity is boosted by stress) appear to increase the degree to which the comparator selects items (originating from neocortical sensory systems via the entorhinal area) for processing; it is in this way that they increase anxiety. Conversely, the anti-anxiety drugs reduce anxiety by limiting the degree to which these monoaminergic inputs enhance the capacity of the comparator to process information, thus impairing both checking behaviour and the consequent detection of mismatch or the threat of mismatch.

Figure 2 illustrates the psychological functions that must be discharged for such a comparator to work; it can be regarded as a flow-chart of the main 'software' of anxiety. The 'hardware' that instantiates this software is presented diagrammatically in figure 3, with tentative labels attaching particular functions (e.g. the comparator function itself) to particular pathways or regions (e.g. the subicular area) [for details, see *Gray*, 1982a]. Note that this approach to the psychology of anxiety has come up with a distinctively cognitive theory of its subject matter. This is not altogether surprising, since cognitive processes are necessarily conducted in the brain, and it is by way of an analysis of brain function that the theory has been constructed. But somehow cognitive processes must eventuate in behaviour and in the signs and symptoms of anxiety that the physician observes. So we must next ask; 'How does the system displayed in figure 3 affect the organism in which it is housed?'

In answering this question – and again I must be dogmatic, relying on previous publications [*Gray*, 1982a, b] – it is useful to refer back to the outputs illustrated to the right of figure 1. (This figure can now be seen as an earlier 'behaviourist' version of the more fully developed and more cognitive theory shown in figure 3.)

The inhibition of ongoing behaviour that is such a prominent feature of anxiety is most likely mediated by projections that link the septo-hippocampal system (by way of the subicular area) to the basal ganglia and cingulate cortex; a further possible route is provided by afferents to the hypothalamus descending from the septal area. In either event, the inhibition of behaviour is not a direct blockade of motor systems, but seems rather to be executed at the level of programs for action, which are interrupted by messages from the comparator system. There is possibly a difference between the subiculo-cingulate and septo-hypothalamic projections, with the former interrupting learned motor programs and the latter innate ones. The serotonergic projection to the septohippocampal and other systems appears to facilitate the inhibition of motor programs [*Williams and Azmitia*, 1981].

The increased attention shown as a second output of the behavioural inhibition system (fig. 1) is an integral part of the software depicted in figure 2. Heightened activity in the comparator necessarily requires increased neocortical sensory input via the entorhinal area. Under conditions of mismatch this process probably comes under the direct control of the septo-hippocampal system (allowing selection of significant items for checking) via the projection from the subiculum to the entorhinal cortex (fig. 3). Selection of items for checking is further enhanced (as noted above) by the ascending monoaminergic inputs to the septo-hippocampal system, especially the noradrenergic afferents from the locus coeruleus [*McNaughton and Mason*, 1980].

Two other features of anxiety appear not to involve the septo-hippocampal system directly but to depend upon the activation of other noradrenergic projections from the locus coeruleus [*Redmond*, 1979]. The first is the increased readiness for rapid and vigorous action which occurs concurrently with increased behavioural inhibition (and which may be masked by the latter) – i.e. the 'increased arousal' of figure 1. This feature of anxiety appears to reflect a rather general effect of locus coeruleus projections throughout the brain, However, a particularly important role is probably played by the projection to the hypothalamus, in which action patterns for innate emotional behavioural routines appear to be stored [*Panksepp*, 1982]. Noradrenergic projections to the hypothalamus from other brain-stem nuclei besides the locus coeruleus may also play a part in elevating arousal.

The remaining feature of anxiety is often particularly prominent clinically, yet it has so far not been mentioned here and does not even appear as one of the outputs of the behavioural inhibition system depicted in figure 1. This feature consists of the well-known autonomic signs of anxiety (cardiovascular, respiratory, electrodermal, etc.) [*Lader*, 1975]. Its absence from figure 1 carries no deep significance; it is due simply to the fact that the animal experiments which form the data base for that figure have almost never included measurements of such autonomic responses. However, data summarised by *Redmond* [1979], in an impressive and wide-ranging review of the neurology of anxiety, allow an easy integration between this feature of anxiety and the others considered already: the autonomic signs of anxiety appear to be mediated largely by efferents from the locus coeruleus that descend into the spinal cord. There is evidence that such autonomic responses are susceptible to blockade by opiate drugs, probably acting upon opiate receptors in the locus coeruleus [*Redmond*, 1979]. This effect of the opiates contrasts with their failure to exert anxiolytic-like action in well-validated behavioural tests of anxiety [*Geller* et al., 1963]. I have considered this problem elsewhere and suggested a possible solution [*Gray*, in press].

This discussion of the neurology of anxiety took as its starting point the action of anti-anxiety drugs. However, some patients fail to respond to these drugs or any other method of treatment. In such cases, a treatment of last resort is provided by psychosurgery. Both prefrontal leucotomy and damage to the cingulate cortex have been shown to reduce anxiety in patients who have suffered severely for many years and who have failed to benefit from either pharmacological or other treatments [for a review, see *Powell*, 1979]. Further elaboration of the theory of anxiety outlined here is clearly necessary to take account of such drug-resistant anxiety disorders and the role played in them by the prefrontal and cingulate cortices. This elaboration [*Gray*, 1982a] has taken the form of attributing to the prefrontal cortex a role in establishing control over the functioning of the septo-hippocampal comparator by verbal systems located in the language areas of the neocortex. The route by which such prefrontal control is exerted includes projections to the cingulate and entorhinal areas. According to the theory, control of the comparator by language systems, exercised by this route, is of particular importance in cases in which the source of threat has become largely internalised (e.g. in the form of verbally formulated standards of behaviour that an obsessive patient attempts to meet). It is patients of this kind who appear to benefit most from psychosurgery.

The Neurology of Depression

The brain mechanisms that mediate depression are less well understood than those that mediate anxiety. There are several reasons for this. First, there is still confusion clinically as to whether depression is a unitary condition varying principally in severity or whether it can be subdivided; and, if subdivision is possible, it is still uncertain whether this should be carried out categorically or by ranking patients and/or symptoms along one or more continua [for a discussion of these problems, see *Roth*, 1979]. Second, almost equally plausible cases can be made for the views that anti-depressant drugs (tricyclics and monoamine oxidase inhibitors) act by *increasing* or *decreasing* net monoaminergic (and perhaps especially noradrenergic) synaptic transmission [*Stone*, 1983]. (Notice that on the former view anti-depressants act in the opposite manner to anti-anxiety drugs, but on the latter view they act in the same manner. This might then imply either that depression is the opposite of anxiety or that it is the same condition as anxiety. If there are two different kinds of depression, the former inference would apply well to 'psychotic' depression, the latter to 'neurotic' depression. These amblyopic complexities are discussed in detail by *Gray* [1982a].) Finally, there are no clear-cut behavioural tests of depression in animals which might allow the construction for depression of a model equivalent to that shown for anxiety in figure 1.

The research which has so far come closest to providing such tests is related to the concept of 'learned helplessness' [*Seligman*, 1975]. If an animal is exposed to uncontrollable aversive stimuli (e.g. footshock, forced swimming in cold water) and is then given an opportunity to avoid or escape from such stimuli, there is observed an impairment in the animal's ability to carry out appropriate avoidance or escape behaviour relative to controls initially exposed to controllable or no aversive stimuli. This is the basic phenomenon termed by *Seligman* [1975] as 'learned helplessness'; however, since there is considerable controversy as to whether the observed behaviour in fact reflects any learning [*Weiss* et al., 1976], it is safer to term it simply 'helplessness'.

Several arguments support the relevance of helplessness in animals to human depression. There is evidence that, in both conditions, lack of control over aversive events is an important precipitating factor, and that inability to exercise control even when it is possible to do so is an important symptom [*Seligman*, 1975]. A more wide-ranging similarity of symptoms of the two conditions has been noted by *Weiss* et al. [1982] and is reproduced here as table I. Pharmacological data, showing that helplessness in animals can be reversed selectively by anti-depressants, have been adduced by *Sherman and Petty* [1982]. Further, *Weiss's* group [Weiss et al., 1976, 1982] have demonstrated an important role in helplessness in the rat of the same noradrenergic mechanisms that have been implicated in human depression [*Van Praag,* 1978]. However, there is a major problem in integrating these diverse strands of evidence into a single coherent story: there is almost certainly more than one kind of helplessness in animals, and the evidence summarised above does not all relate to the same kind.

The demonstration that helplessness comes in more than one form comes from *Glazer and Weiss* [1976]. These workers showed, in rats, that exposure to high-intensity, short-duration, uncontrollable shock gives rise to a form of helplessness that is closely related to changes in the levels of noradrenaline in the brain, whereas exposure to low-intensity, long-duration, uncontrollable shock gives rise to helplessness that appears not to relate closely to noradrenergic mechanisms in the brain. The two forms of helplessness differed also in other ways: 'noradrenergic' helplessness was of shorter duration than 'non-noradrenergic' helplessness (so that *Glazer and Weiss* called the two phenomena 'short-term' and 'long-term' interference effects, respectively); and *prolonged* initial exposure to uncontrollable shock caused helplessness to disappear (an effect termed 'toughening up') in the case of noradrenergic but not non-noradrenergic helplessness. (We shall return to the phenomenon of toughening up in the final section of this chapter.) Given the relevance of noradrenergic mechanisms to human depression [*Stone,* 1983], it is *Weiss's* short-term interference effect that one is tempted to relate to the clinical condition. To be able to make this step with any confidence, however, we would need to know which form of helplessness responds to anti-depressant medication. Unfortunately, *Sherman and Petty* [1982], who have provided most of the pharmacological data, have used their own behavioural paradigm and this cannot (in the absence of relevant experiments) be aligned with either *Weiss's* short-term or long-term interference effect.

If we nonetheless assume for the moment that *Weiss's* short-term, noradrenergic interference effect is a model for human depression, we come up against two other intractable problems.

First, though it seems clear that the short-term interference effect depends in some manner on changes in noradrenergic transmission, it is uncertain whether these changes give rise to an increase or a decrease in

Table I. Comparison of the effects of uncontrollable shock with symptomatic indications of depression from the third edition of the Diagnostic and Statistical Manual for Mental Disorders (DSM-III).

Uncontrollable shock as a model of depression		DSM-III criteria for depression: four of the following
Uncontrollable shock produces the following symptomatology		
1. Decreased food and/or water consumption	Brady, Thornton, and Fisher, 1962 [ref. 17] Pare, 1964 [18] Pare, 1965 [19] * Weiss, 1968 [12] Ritter, Pelzer, and Ritter, 1978 [13]	1. poor appetite and significant weight loss
2. Weight loss	Brady, Thornton, and Fisher, 1962 [17] Pare, 1965 [19] * Weiss, 1968 [12]	2. psychomotor alterations
3. Poor performance in tasks requiring active motor behaviour (Shuttle advoidance-escape, lever-press escape, water-escape, open-field activity, etc.)	Overmier and Seligman, 1967 [1] *Seligman and Maier, 1967 [2] Overmier, 1968 [20] Weiss and Glazer, 1975 [11] Weiss, Glazer, Pohorecky, Brick, and Miller, 1975 [21] Weiss, Bailey, Korzeniowski, and Grillone, 1980 [22] * Weiss, Goodman, Losito, Corrigan, Harry, and Bailey, 1981 [15] * Sutton, Coover, and Lints, 1981 [23]	3. loss of energy or fatigue 4. loss of interst in usual activities 5. sleep changes

noradrenergic transmission (the same ambiguity that clouds current understanding of the mode of action of anti-depressant drugs).

The data reported by *Weiss's* group in 1975 suggested that noradrenergic transmission was decreased in animals made helpless by high-intensity uncontrollable shock. Whole-brain levels of noradrenaline were lowered in such animals at the time that they displayed behavioural

Table I. (cont.)

Uncontrollable shock as a model of depression		DSM-III criteria for depression: four of the following
4. Loss of normal aggressiveness or competitiveness	Peters and Finch, 1961 [24] * Maier, Anderson, and Leiberman, 1972 [25] * Corum and Thurmond, 1977 [26]	6. indecisiveness, evidence of decreased ability to think
5. Loss of normal grooming or play activity	* Redmond, Maas, Dekirmanjian, and Schlemmer, 1973 [27] Stone, 1980 [14] * Weiss, Goodman, Losito, Corrigan, Harry, and Bailley, 1981 [15]	7. *Feelings* of worth-lessness
6. Decreased sleep	* Weiss, Goodman, Losito, Corrigan, Harry and Bailey, 1981 – unpubl. observation [16]	8. Recurrent *thoughts* of death and suicide

For references in this table see *Weiss* et al. [1982].
* Denotes study demonstrating that the effect depends on uncontrollability of shock

helplessness; and prolonged exposure to uncontrollable shock, causing toughening up, eliminated the fall in noradrenaline levels, apparently by increasing the activity of tyrosine hydroxylase, the rate-limiting enzyme in the synthesis of noradrenaline. This pattern of results was consistent with the hypothesis that helplessness was due to a reduction in the availability of noradrenaline for release at neuronal terminals.

However, subsequent research [*Weiss* et al., 1982] showed that both the fall in noradrenaline levels due to exposure to uncontrollable shock, and the subsequent rise in noradrenaline levels with prolongation of this exposure (together with increased activity of tyrosine hydroxylase), were confined to the region of the locus coeruleus and did not occur in terminal regions of the locus coeruleus projection. *Weiss* et al. [1982] interpret these findings in the light of the presence on locus coeruleus cell bodies of alpha-adrenergic auto-receptors, that is, receptors which, when stimulated by noradrenaline released by local recurrent collaterals, act to inhibit further firing of noradrenergic axons destined for the forebrain. Their hypothesis now supposes that, during helplessness, there is a reduction in stimulation of these auto-receptors (consequent upon lowered availability of noradrenaline) and so an *increase* in the activity of noradrenergic terminals in the forebrain. In short, far from helplessness reflecting lowered noradrenergic transmission as in the 1975 hypothesis, it now reflects increased noradrenergic transmission.

The second problem that we must face in interpreting *Weiss's* findings is this: supposing that the short-term interference effect is a model of some kind of depression, and supposing also that there is more than one kind of depression, is it a model of psychotic or neurotic depression? *Weiss* et al. [1975] believed that they were studying a model of psychotic depression, and this view is supported by the symptoms gathered together in table I. However, now that their data have forced them to the hypothesis that helplessness reflects an increase in forebrain noradrenergic transmission, they prefer the view that they have a model of neurotic depression, i.e. the form of depression that is closest to (and perhaps identical with) anxiety [*Roth*, 1979]. Again, pharmacological data, of the kind gathered by *Sherman and Petty* but using *Weiss's* short-term interference effect, might resolve this problem.

Having indicated all the complexities and possibilities for double vision in this field [see also *Gray* 1982a; *Stone*, 1984], I shall now indicate my own view of the data. If we assume, with *Weiss* et al. [1982], that their short-term interference effect is due to increased forebrain noradrenaline release, and if we take into account the analysis of the neurology of anxiety with which this chapter began, then we must conclude (again with *Weiss* et al. [1982]) that the short-term interference effect is a model of either anxiety or something very close to anxiety (since anxiety too depends on increased release of noradrenaline). This leaves open the possibility that *Weiss's* long-term interference effect (and *Seligman's* original observation of helplessness in animals, which rather resembles the long-term than the short-term interference effect) is a model of psychotic depression. But since we know nothing of the neurology of the long-term interference effect, this tells us nothing of the neurology of depression. In short, we are left with the neurology of anxiety as outlined in the first section of this chapter, now supplemented by the very interesting data reported by *Weiss* et al. [1975, 1982]. Whether this is the neurology of anxiety, of neurotic depression or of both depends upon a prior judgement as to whether these two conditions truly differ; my own view is that they do not, but that psychotic depression is different from both [*Gray,* 1982a].

The Neurology of Tolerance for Stress

As noted in the previous section, the behavioural effects of exposure to uncontrollable footshock or cold swims or other such aversive events vary with the duration of exposure. Exposure on relatively few occasions disrupts behaviour, but exposure on many occasions eliminates the disruption. As an example (but there are many others), *Weiss* et al. [1975] found that rats tested in a two-compartment apparatus (a 'shuttlebox') in which they could escape from shock by jumping from side to side behaved differently depending on whether they had previously been exposed to a single session of uncontrollable footshock or to 15 daily sessions of this kind. In the former case, they were unable to escape the shock when tested in the shuttlebox, in the latter they were like unshocked controls. As we also saw, this 'toughening-up' effect of prolonged exposure to uncontrollable shock is apparently due to changes in the capacity of noradrenergic neurons to synthesis their transmitter, noradrenaline [*Weiss* et al., 1982]. Given the conclusion, reached in the previous section, that the initial disruption of shuttlebox performance studied by *Weiss's* group is probably related to anxiety, it is natural to ask whether the brain systems responsible for anxiety are involved also in the development of tolerance for repeated stress.

Evidence that this is indeed the case comes from a series of experiments in my own laboratory. These experiments have employed tasks which, while differing from those used by *Weiss's* group in many respects, have in common the feature that the animal's tolerance for events that normally disrupt behaviour is increased by exposure to those events. Two phenomena in particular have engaged much of our attention – the partial punishment effect (PPE) and the partial reinforcement extinction effect (PREE). Both of these phenomena are observed in a straight alley which the rat has to traverse to obtain, in the goalbox, a food reward. Three basic training schedules are used. The first, a continuous reinforcement (CRF) schedule, involves simply the delivery of the food reward on each occasion (a trial) that the rat runs down the alley. The second, a partial punishment (PP) schedule, adds to the food reward a footshock delivered on a randomly chosen 50% of trials just as the rat enters the goalbox and just before it takes the food. The third, a partial reinforcement (PRF) schedule, employs no shock, but omits the food reward on a randomly chosen 50% of trials. (This is the event of nonreward, which we encountered in the discussion of the behavioural inhibition system depicted in figure 1. The stressful nature of nonreward is demonstrated by its capacity to elicit a rise in plasma corticosterone, [*Goldman* et al., 1973].) The PPE consists in the fact that, if animals initially trained on CRF and PP schedules are tested with food and shock given on every trial (continuous punishment), the PP-trained animals show more resistance to punishment (that is, they continue to run to the goalbox for longer and run faster) than the CRF-trained animals. Similarly, the PREE consists in the fact that, if CRF- and PRF-trained animals are tested with nonreward on every trial (an extinction schedule), the PRF animals show more resistance to extinction than CRF animals. That these two phenomena share common mechanisms is suggested by the demonstration [*Brown and Wagner*, 1964] of cross-tolerance between them: that is, animals trained on a PRF schedule display increased resistance to punishment and animals trained on a PP schedule display increased resistance to extinction, in both cases relative to animals trained on CRF.

The first indication that the brain systems mediating these phenomena might be related to those that mediate anxiety came from the demonstration that, under certain conditions, both the PPE [*Davis* et al., 1981] and the PREE [*Gray*, 1969; *Feldon* et al., 1979; *Feldon and Gray*, 1981] are abolished if animals are trained after administration of an anxiolytic dose of a barbiturate or a benzodiazepine. Given the general evidence, outlined earlier in this chapter, that anxiety is a function of the septo-hippocampal system, we followed up these findings by investigating the effects of damage to this system on the PREE and PPE. While initially our experiments yielded evidence that strongly supported a role for the septo-hippocampal system in the PREE [*Gray* et al., 1978], our most recent findings show that this role is constrained by temporal parameters that are clearly different from those that determine the effects of the anti-anxiety drugs [*Rawlins*, in press]. In other experiments we have demonstrated a role in behavioural tolerance for stress for the ascending noradrenergic (but not serotonergic) fibres that innervate the septo-hippocampal system [*Owen* et al., 1982; *Davis and Gray*, 1983; *Tsaltas and Gray*, in preparation]. Again, however, the parameters that constrain the effects of lesions to the dorsal noradrenergic bundle (carrying the ascending noradrenergic efferents from the locus coeruleus) differ from those that constrain the effects of anxiolytic drugs, resembling rather the parameters applicable to damage to the septo-hippocampal system [*Owen* et al., 1982; *Tsaltas and Gray*, in preparation; *Gray and McNaughton*, 1983]. Thus, present data from lesion experiments permit the conclusion that the septo-hippocampal system and its noradrenergic afferents are in some way involved in the development of tolerance for stress, but fail to indicate a clear mechanism for the action of anti-anxiety drugs in blocking the development of such stress tolerance.

Further evidence for the involvement of the septo-hippocampal system in the development of tolerance for stress comes from experiments in which we have, via chronically implanted electrodes, stimulated the septal area in conscious rats. It is well known that the medial septal area contains the pacemaker cells that control (via a diffuse cholinergic projection travelling in the fornix and fimbria) the slow, high-voltage electrical waves in the hippocampal formation known as the 'theta rhythm' [for a review, see *Gray*, 1982a]. If one stimulates the septal area using short (ca. 0.5 ms) pulses at a frequency lying within the natural theta range (6–12 Hz in the rat) one can artificially drive the hippocampal theta rhythm at the imposed frequency. We have recently shown that a course of ten days' stimulation of this kind (a total of 90 s of stimulation per day) alters the rat's behaviour several weeks later in a manner that is consistent with the hypothesis that the animal has been rendered behaviourally more tolerant of stress. Relative to unstimulated controls the stimulated rats show more resistance to extinction, to punishment and to disruption of responding (pressing a bar for food reward) by stimuli associated with footshock [*Holt and Gray*, 1983a, in press]. These results are obtained even though the barpressing response is not acquired until the period of septal stimulation is over.

These intriguing findings suggest that septal stimulation in some way mimics the neural consequences of exposure to aversive stimuli (though the stimulation is not aversive in its own right) [*Ball and Gray* , 1971]. We cannot yet be sure that the critical feature of the stimulation is its driving of the hippocampal theta rhythm, but several findings clearly point in this direction. First, if high-frequency electrical stimulation is applied to the septal area, this disrupts rather than drives the theta rhythm; such stimulation proactively reduces resistance to extinction [*Holt and Gray*, 1983b] – the opposite effect to that observed after theta-driving stimulation. Second, the frequency of septal stimulation that increases tolerance for stress is 7.7 Hz [*Gray*, 1972]. This is an important finding, since anti-anxiety drugs raise the threshold for septal driving of hippocampal theta selectively at this same frequency of 7.7 Hz [*McNaughton* et al., 1977]. Thus, the *increase* in tolerance for stress produced by septal stimulation appears to depend upon *activation* of the same mechanism (i.e., an input to the hippocampal formation eliciting 7.7-Hz theta) which is *blocked* by anti-anxiety drugs when they *reduce* tolerance for stress.

Resistance to Cancer

Now, the latter effect – elevation of the threshold for 7.7-Hz theta driving by anxiolytic drugs – is almost certainly due to a reduction in the noradrenergic input to the septo-hippocampal system from the locus coeruleus [*Gray* et al., 1975; *McNaughton* et al., 1977]. Thus, one might perhaps expect the increased tolerance for stress caused by repeated 7.7-Hz theta driving to be accompanied by signs of increased noradrenergic input to the septo-hippocampal system. We have indeed observed such signs. After the same regime of septal stimulation that produces increased tolerance for stress there is increased activity of tyrosine hydroxylase in the hippocampus [*Graham-Jones* et al., in press]. This finding is reminiscent of the report by *Weiss's* group that the regime of exposure to uncontrollable footshock which gave rise to behavioural toughening up was accompanied by increased tyrosine hydroxylation in the brain. However, as noted in the previous section, this biochemical change was confined to the region of the cell bodies in the locus coeruleus [*Weiss* et al., 1982]. The significance of this discrepancy in the location of the increased activity of tyrosine hydroxylase in the two sets of experiments is at present unclear. But both sets of experiments concur in suggesting that increased activity of the rate-limiting enzyme in noradrenaline synthesis, i.e. tyrosine hydroxylase, may contribute to the development of behavioural tolerance for stress.

The central concern of this book is with psychosomatic medicine. However, the role of the brain in psychosomatic disorders is still very obscure [*Fauman*, 1982]. It is for this reason that I have confined my attention to more general issues related to the role of the brain in emotion and reactions to stress. Nonetheless, it is perhaps appropriate to bring this chapter to a close with an attempt – no matter how speculative – to relate behavioural tolerance for stress to a classic psychosomatic problem: resistance to cancer.

The role of psychological factors in the progress of human cancers is now well established, as is the corresponding role of stress and behavioural factors in cancers in animals [*Riley*, 1981; *Sklar and Anisman*, 1981]. For our present purpose, one particular feature of the experiments with animals demands attention. Recall that, in *Weiss's* experiments, it was shown that exposure to a single session of uncontrollable (but not controllable) shock disrupted subsequent behaviour in the shuttlebox, whereas exposure to repeated sessions of uncontrollable shock eliminated this behavioural disruption. *Anisman's* group, working with mice, has demonstrated a closely similar pattern of change in the rate of growth of cancer cells: a single session of uncontrollable (but not controllable) shock causes experimentally induced tumours to grow faster, whereas repeated shock sessions causes them to grow slower [*Sklar and Anisman,* 1981].

These observations suggest that the same brain mechanisms that mediate the development of behavioural tolerance for stress may also mediate resistance to cancer. If this is so, and if it is correct (as argued above) to implicate the septo-hippocampal system and ascending noradrenergic fibres in behavioural tolerance for stress, then it is possible that these structures also play a role in determining resistance to cancer. We are currently investigating this hypothesis, by measuring the rate of tumour growth in animals that have previously been subjected to septal driving of the hippocampal theta rhythm. If one may extrapolate from our earlier behavioural observations [*Holt and Gray,* 1983a], such stimulation should retard the growth of a tumour implanted after the period of stimulation is over. Such an outcome of our experiments is, of course, inherently unlikely; but it would not be without parallel, since there is already evidence that lesions to the brain (principally the hypothalamus, with which the septal area has intimate reciprocal connections) can affect the immune system [*Fauman,* 1982].

Conclusion

The role played by the brain in the control of emotional behaviour is still obscure, but islands of clarity are beginning to emerge. The structures that mediate anxiety (at least some of them) have been marked out, and their function in processing information is yielding to analysis. Although the major advances in our understanding of the neuropsychology of anxiety have come from animal experiments, recent observations on patients suffering from panic disorder (using the new brain imaging technique of positron emission tomography) have confirmed the importance of the hippocampal formation and its connections with the temporal lobe [*Reiman* et al., 1984]. There is evidence that the structures concerned with the development of tolerance for stress are closely related to those that mediate anxiety. The hippocampus (once more) and other systems connected to it have been demonstrated in several experiments from my own laboratory to play a key role in determining behavioural tolerance for stress. It is interesting to note that this structure contains many of the physiological elements found also in peripheral systems involved in stress responding: cholinergic and noradrenergic afferent pathways, and cells that avidly bind adrenocortical hormones [*McEwen* et al., 1969]. Thus, it may yet turn out that the principles that govern the role of peripheral structures in responding to stress are applicable also to the central nervous system. But much experimental work remains to be done before we can see these (or any other) principles at all clearly.

References

Ball, G.G.; Gray, J.A.: Septal self-stimulation and hippocampal activity. Physiol. Behav. *6:* 547–549 (1971).

Bowery, N.G.: Actions and interactions of GABA and benzodiazepines (Raven Press, New York 1984).

Braestrup, C.; Squires, R.F.: Specific benzodiazepine receptors in rat brain characterized by high-affinity (^{3}H)-diazepam binding. Proc. natn. Acad. Sci. USA *90:* 694–703 (1977).

Brown, R.T.; Wagner, A.R.: Resistance to punishment and extinction following training with shock or non-reinforcement. J. exp. Psychol. *68:* 503–507 (1964).

Costa, E.: The benzodiazepines: from molecular biology to clinical practice (Raven Press, New York 1983).

Davis, N.M.; Brookes, S.; Gray, J.A.; Rawlins, J.N.P.: Chlordiazepoxide and resistance to punishment. Q. Jl exp. Psychol. *33B:* 227–239 (1981).

Davis, N.M.; Gray, J.A.: Brain 5-hydroxytryptamine and learned resistance to punishment. Behav. Brain Res. *8:* 129–137 (1983).

Elliot, K.; Whelan, J.: Functions of the septo-hippocampal system. Ciba Foundation Symp. No. 58 (New Series), pp. 275–300 (Elsevier, Amsterdam 1978).

Fauman, M.A.: The central nervous system and the immune system. Biol. Psychiat. *17:* 1459–1483 (1982).

Feldon, J.; Gray, J.A.: The partial reinforcement extinction effect after treatment with chlordiazepoxide. Psychopharmacology *73:* 269–275 (1981).

Feldon, J.; Guillamon, A.; Gray, J.A.; De Wit, H.; McNaughton, N.: Sodium amylobarbitone and responses to nonreward. Qt. Jl. exp. Psychol. *296:* 97–98 (1979).

Geller, I.; Bachman, E.; Seifter, J.: Effects of reserpine and morphine on behaviour suppressed by punishment. Life Sci. *4:* 226–231 (1963).

Glazer, H.I.; Weiss, J.M.: Long-term interference effect: an alternative to 'learned helplessness'. J. exp. Psychol. *2:* 202–213 (1976).

Goldman, L.; Coover, G.D.; Levine, S.: Bidirectional effects of reinforcement shifts on pituitary adrenal activity. Physiol. Behav. *10:* 209–214 (1973).

Graham-Jones, S.; Holt, L.; Gray, J.A.; Fillenz, M.: Low-frequency septal stimulation increases tyrosine hydroxylase activity in the hippocampus. Pharmacol. Biochem. Behav. (in press, 1985).

Gray, J.A.: Sodium amobarbital and effects of frustrative non-reward. J. comp. Physiol. Psychol. *69:* 55–64 (1969).

Gray, J.A.: Effects of septal driving of the hippocampal theta rhythm on resistance to extinction. Physiol. Behav. *8:* 481–490 (1972).

Gray, J.A.: Drug effects on fear and frustration: possible limbic site of action of minor tranquilizers; in Iversen, Iversen, Snyder, Handbook of phsychopharmacology, vol 8, pp. 433–529 (Plenum Press, New York 1977).

Gray, J.A.: The neuropsychology of anxiety: an enquiry into the function of the septo-hippocampal system (Oxford University Press, Oxford 1982a).

Gray, J.A.: Précis of 'The neuropsychology of anxiety: an enquiry into the functions of the septo-hippocampal system'. Behav. Brain Sci. *5:* 469–484 (1982b).

Gray, J.A.: Issues in the neuropsychology of anxiety; in Maser, Anxiety and the anxiety disorders (Lawrence Erlbaum Associates, in press).

Gray, J.A.; Feldon, J.; Rawlins, J.N.P.; Owen, S.; McNaughton, N.: The role of the septo-hippocampal system and its noradrenergic afferents in behavioural responses to nonreward; in Elliott, Whelan, Functions of the septo-hippocampal system. Ciba Foundation Symp. No. 58 (New Series), pp. 275–300 (Elsevier, Amsterdam 1978).

Gray, J.A.; McNaughton, N.: Comparison between the behavioural effects of septal and hippocampal lesions. A review. Neurosci. Biobehav. Rev. *7:* 119–188 (1983).

Gray, J.A.; McNaughton, N.; James, D.T.D.; Kelly, P.H.: Effect of minor tranquilisers on hippocampal theta rhythm mimicked by depletion of forebrain noradrenaline. Nature, Lond. *258:* 424–425 (1976).

Gray, J.A.; Quintero, S.; Mellanby, J.; Buckland, C.; Fillenz, M.; Fung, S.C.: Some biochemical, behavioural and electrophysiological tests of the GABA hypothesis of anti-anxiety drug action; in Bowery, Actions and interactions of GABA and benzodiazepines, pp. 239–262 (Raven Press, New York 1984).

Holt, L.; Gray, J.A.: Septal driving of the hippocampal theta rhythm produces a long-term, proactive and non-associative increase in resistance to extinction. Q. Jl exp. Psychol. *35B:* 97–118 (1983a).

Holt, L.; Gray, J.A.: Proactive behavioral effects of theta-blocking septal stimulation in the rat. Behav. neural Biol. *39:* 7–21 (1983b).

Holt, L.; Gray, J.A.: Proactive behavioural effects of theta-driving septal stimulation on conditioned suppression and punishment in the rat. Behav. Neurosci. (In press, 1984).

Isaacson, R.L.: The limbic system (Plenum Press, New York 1974).

Lader, M.H.: The psychophysiology of mental illness (Routledge & Kegan, London 1975).

Lidbrink, P.; Corrodi, H.; Fuxe, K.; Olson, L.: Barbiturates and meprobamate: decreases in catecholamine turnover of central dopamine and noradrenaline neuronal systems and the influence of immobilization stress. Brain Res. *45:* 507–524 (1972).

McEwen, B.S.; Weiss, J.M.; Schwartz, L.S.: Uptake of corticosterone by rat brain and its concentration by certain limbic structures. Brain Res. *16:* 227–241 (1969).

McNaughton, N.; James, D.T.D.; Stewart, J.; Gray, J.A.; Valero, I.; Drewnowski, A.: Septal driving of hippocampal theta rhythm as a function of frequency in the male rat: effects of drugs. Neuroscience *2:* 1019–1027 (1977).

McNaughton, N.; Mason, S.T.: The neuropsychology and neuropharmacology of the dorsal ascending noradrenergic bundle – a review. Prog. Neurobiol. *14:* 157–219 (1980).

Möhler, H.; Okada, T.: Benzodiazepine receptor: demonstration in the central nervous system. Science, N.Y. *198:* 849–851 (1977).

Nielsen, M.; Braestrup, C.; Squires, R.F.: Evidence for a late evolutionary appearance of brain-specific benzodiazepine receptors: an investigation of 18 vertebrate and 5 invertebrate species. Brain Res. *141:* 342–346 (1978).

Olsen, R.W.: GABA-benzodiazepine-barbiturate receptor interactions. J. Neurochem. *37:* 1–13 (1981).

Owen, S.; Boarder, M.; Gray, J.A.; Fillenz, M.: Acquisition and extinction of continuously and partially reinforced running in rats with lesions of the dorsal noradrenergic bundle. Behav. Brain Res. *5:* 11–41 (1982).

Panksepp, J.: Toward a general psychological theory of emotions. Behav. Brain Sci. *5:* 407–467 (1982).

Papez, J.W.; A proposed mechanism of emotion. Archs Neurol. Psychiat. *38:* 725–743 (1937).

Powell, G.E.: Brain and personality (Saxon House, London 1979).

Rawlins, J.N.P.: Associations across time: the hippocampus as a temporary memory store. Behav. Brain Sci. (in press).

Redmond, D.E. Jr.: New and old evidence for the involvement of a brain norepinephrine system in anxiety; in Fann, Karacan, Pokorny, Williams, Phenomenology and treatment of anxiety, pp. 153–203 (Spectrum, New York 1979).

Reiman, E.M.; Raichle, M.E.; Butler, F.K.; Herscovitch, P.; Robins, E.: Positron emission tomography demonstrates a focal brain abnormality in panic disorders. 14th Congr. collegium Int. Neuro-Psychopharmacologicum, Florence 1984.

Rickels, K.: Use of anti-anxiety agents in anxious outpatients. Psychopharmacology *58:* 1–17 (1978).

Riley, V.: Psychoneuroendocrine influences on immunocompetence and neoplasia. Science *212:* 1100–1109 (1981).

Roth, M.: A classification of affective disorders based on a synthesis of new and old concepts; in Meyer, Brady, Research in the psychobiology of human behaviour, pp. 75–114 (Johns Hopkins University Press, Baltimore 1979).

Segal, M.: The effects of brainstem priming stimulation on interhemispheric hippocampal responses in the awake rat. Exp. Brain Res. *28:* 529–541 (1977).

Seligman, M.E.P.: Helplessness (Freeman, San Francisco 1975).

Sherman, A.D.; Petty, F.: Specificity of the learned helplessness animal model of depression. Pharmac. Biochem. Behav. *16:* 449–454 (1982).

Sklar, L.S.; Anisman, H.: Stress and cancer. Psychol. Bull. *89:* 369–406 (1981).

Stone, E.A.: Problems with current catecholamine hypotheses of antidepressant agents. Behav. Brain Sci. *6:* 535–577 (1983).

Van Praag, H.M.: Amine hypotheses of affective disorders; in Iversen, Iversen, Snyder, Biology of mood and antianxiety drugs. Handbook of psychopharmacology, 13, pp. 187–297 (Plenum Press, New York 1978).

Weiss, J.M.; Bailey, W.H.; Goodman, P.A.; Hoffman, L.J.; Ambrose, M.J.; Salman, S.; Charry, J.M.: A model for neurochemical study of depression; in Spiegelstein, Levy, Behavioral models and the analysis of drug action (Elsevier, Amsterdam 1982).

Weiss, J.M.; Glazer, H.I.; Pohorecky, L.A.: Coping behavior and neurochemical changes: an alternative explanation for the original 'learned helplessness' experiments; in Serban, Kling, Animal models in human psychobiology, pp. 141–173 (Plenum Press, New York 1976).

Weiss, J.M.; Glazer, H.I.; Pohorecky, L.A.; Brick, J.; Miller, N.E.: Effects of chronic exposure to stressors on avoidance-escape behavior and on brain norepinephrine. Psychosom. Med. *37:* 522–534 (1975).

Williams, J.H.; Azmitia, E.C.: Hippocampal serotonin reuptake and nocturnal locomotor activity after microinjections of 5,7-DHT in the fornix-fimbria. Brain Res. *207:* 95–107.

J.A. Gray, PhD, Department of Psychology, Institute of Psychiatry,
De Crespigny Park, Denmark Hill, London SE55 8AF (UK)

2. The Social Environment and Neurological Disease[1]

Igor Grant[2]

University of California, San Diego and San Diego VA, Medical Center, La Jolla, Calif., USA

Both common observation and systematic research indicate that the social environment can, under certain circumstances, exert a deleterious effect on people's health. Most of the research has been conducted with psychiatric and general medical problems; nevertheless, there is a small but growing literature concerning neurological afflictions as well. In this chapter, research concerned with psychosocial influences on three common neurological diseases –, epilepsy, stroke, and multiple sclerosis – will be reviewed. To put these studies into context, it is necessary first to consider some of the methodological and theoretical issues in research which attempts to link aspects of the social environment to health.

Some Definitions

The term social environment is a broad one, encompassing as it does transactions which range from one-to-one relationships to those between an individual and various social systems. For research purposes it has been convenient to partition this environment into two major categories: (1) life events and difficulties, and (2) social support networks.

Life events can be defined as occurrences which call for some adaptive response or readjustment on the part of a person. Events can be further

---

[1] This work was supported in part by award MRIS 3240 to Dr. *Igor Grant* from the Medical Research Service of the Veterans Administration.

[2] The author gratefully acknowledges the help of Dr. *Tom Patterson* and Ms. *Jamie Clopton* who assisted in the literature review, and Ms. *Joanne McCoy,* who prepared the manuscript.

classified according to some of their qualitative features. Examples of these qualitative descriptors include extent to which an event can be seen as threatening [*Brown and Harris,* 1978], desirable or undesirable [*Grant* et al., 1981], controllable or uncontrollable [*Grant* et al., 1981], or 'entrance' or 'exit' from the social field [*Paykel* et al., 1969]. One can also consider the 'focus' of an event, that is, whether the occurrence acts directly on the subject being studied, or on some other person that the subject knows.

Difficulties can be thought of as longer term circumstances which pose a continuing requirement to cope. Unemployment, bad housing conditions, or chronic ill health of a spouse are examples of substantial difficulties. Although in most cases it is easy to separate events from difficulties on the basis that the former occur at a point in time whereas the latter span longer periods of time, it is obvious that some events take time to evolve and may involve complex circumstances. Furthermore, events can cause difficulties in their aftermath. For a more detailed treatment of these issues, readers are referred to the discussions of difficulties by *Brown and Harris* [1978] and hassles by *Lazarus'* group [*Kanner* et al., 1981].

Social supports refers to the extent and quality of a person's interpersonal networks. In this category one can consider the number and frequency of person to person contacts, as well as the qualitative features of the relationships involved. For example, *Brown and Harris* [1978] use the term 'confidant' to describe the person with whom a subject has a particularly deep and meaningful relationship. Further, the nature of the support derived can also be categorized. For example, *Lazarus* and colleagues suggest that most social supports can be classified principally as instrumental (i.e. giving practical help) versus emotional support (i.e. sympathy, understanding, and moral support) [*Folkman and Lazarus,* 1980].

The Relationship of Life Events and Health: State of the Art

In this section some of the findings concerning life events and health will be reviewed briefly, and some of the methodological issues will be highlighted. Since it is only recently that researchers have distinguished between life events and difficulties, in this discussion life events and difficulties will be subsumed under the term life events, unless otherwise stated.

The exploration of the relationship of life events to health has used two general strategies to define study groups. The first of these has involved finding populations which have been subjected to extremely stressful events which, on common sense grounds, would be expected to cause considerable distress and require major readaptation. Such events have included deaths of loved ones, natural disasters (such as floods), combat, immigration, confinement in internment or concentration camps. In general, such extreme environmental stressors tend to be accompanied by increases in morbidity and mortality in the populations exposed to them. This was noted in the aftermath of the Bristol floods [*Bennet,* 1970], among Chinese immigrating to the United States following the Communist revolution of 1949 [*Hinkle,* 1974] among Vietnam era veterans subjected to combat [*Figley,* 1978], and among survivors of bereavement [*Parkes* et al., 1969].

Decrements in health are not uniform after even such stresses, however. For example, among the Chinese Nationalist immigrants, only some subgroups became more symptomatic – others, who seemed to be using coping styles involving more denial, actually reported *improved* health postmigration. Similarly, in many cases the death of spouse does not result in increased symptoms, either psychiatric or physical [*Clayton,* 1979]. Generally speaking, authors conducting this line of research have tended to conclude that what a person 'brings' to the situation (in terms of preexisting coping skills, social support networks, personal health and other resources) may be as important as the occurrence of a severe stressor in predicting subsequent morbidity [for further discussion of this see *Hinkle,* 1974].

The second major approach, to be distinguished from the 'disaster approach' reviewed above, can be described as an effort systematically to catalogue many different kinds of life occurrences and to assign stress or threat ratings to them. This second strategy was spearheaded by *Holmes* and associates, who initially developed an inventory of 43 life events which they termed the Schedule of Recent Experiences (SRE) [*Rahe* et al., 1964]. The SRE was followed by the development of the Social Readjustment Rating Questionnaire (SRRQ) which asked subjects to assign 'readjustment weights' to each of the 43 SRE events, using a readjustment score of 500 for marriage as an anchor point [*Masuda and Holmes,* 1967]. The geometric means of the SRRQ weights from a normative sample were then divided by ten to create the well-known Social Readjustment Rating Scale (SRRS) score which assigns a weight of 50 to marriage and 100 to death of a spouse [*Holmes and Rahe,* 1967]. Using the SRE and SRRS weights *Holmes, Rahe,* and collaborators then proceeded to compute 'life change unit' (LCU) scores for people by noting which of the SRE events were reported during a given time period, assigning an SRRS readjustment weight to each event which occurred, and by summing these scores into a grand total LCU score.

Using this strategy of computing the stressfulness of life events, hundreds of investigators have published articles relating results of SRE research to symptoms and illnesses of various kinds [for review see *Rahe and Arthur,* 1978]. In most instances significant but low order correlations (correlation coefficients in the order of 0.2 and 0.3) were reported.

Soon, investigators began noting serious methodological flaws in this type of research – flaws which have served to raise questions about the interpretability of much of the work done with the SRE. Some of the central criticisms include: (1) that some of the SRE items are worded sufficiently vaguely that one could have little confidence that different people are, in fact, reporting on a similar event; (2) that self report checklists of events are subject to forgetting, denial, or inaccuracy in the timing of the event; (3) that some SRE events could actually be thought of as 'symptoms' rather than 'events' (e.g. marital difficulties) – this raises the issue of criterion contamination, i.e. the predictor and the predicted are one and the same, or, at least overlap substantially; (4) that the range of events being sampled in the SRE is either too restrictive generally, or not appropriate for a given population; and (5) that the SRE lacks predictive validity [for discussions of these issues see *Brown and Harris,* 1978; *Dohrenwend and Dohrenwend,* 1977; *Grant* et al., 1982; *Rabkin and Struening,* 1976].

The last-mentioned point requiries some expansion. It has already been noted that many studies found *associations* between SRE measured events and symptoms of various kinds. Virtually all of these studies were, however, cross-sectional and retrospective in nature. In other words, people were reporting on their health and recollecting their events at the same time. Very few studies have adopted a prospective design which would allow a test of whether events truly *preceded* health change. Those few that have made such an attempt have yielded disappointing results; life events bore virtually no predictive relationship to symptoms or health change [*Grant* et al., 1982].

These various methodological problems led investigators to attempt improvements in ascertaining the occurrence of and describing the qualities of events that might have health implications. One strategy has been to improve the life events inventory using *Holmes and Rahe's* SRE as a starting point. Among the best known of these second generation inventories is the Psychiatric Epidemiology Research Interview (PERI) which developed out of the work of the *Dohrenwends* [*Dohrenwend and Dohrenwend*, 1978, *Herschfeld* et al., 1977]. The principal refinements of the PERI are introduction of an interview mode (thereby allowing probing of reported events), a substantially increased coverage in terms of numbers and types of items, and the possibility to qualify the events in various ways, e.g. desirability, controlability, whether the event was anticipated, and what effect the event had on a person's self-esteem. Although on the face of it the PERI should represent a significant methodological advance, there has not been sufficient research with it to state confidently that this is so.

The other major strategy has evolved out of the work of *Brown* and associates at Bedford College. These investigators developed an Interview Schedule for Events and Difficulties which, both in their hands and in those of several other groups of investigators, has shown considerable promise in predicting health change. Essential features of the ISED are (1) the data are gathered by interviewers who undergo extensive training in strategies of questionning, probing, and follow-up; (2) the interview has structured and open ended features, assuring broad coverage and the opportunity to include unusual or unique circumstances; (3) the interviews are tape recorded so that when the information is finally reduced to written form it can be double checked both by the interviewer and by the supervising investigator; (4) there is a system of 'contextual rating' which means that the research group is given an opportunity to decide whether a reported occurrence qualifies as an event by research standards, and how it should be rated in terms of its level of threat, degree of independence or other features.

Although it is this author's opinion that the Bedford College strategy represents, from a methodological standpoint, the soundest approach to life events research, the disadvantage to this strategy is its time-consuming nature. For example, 2 or more hours may need to be spent with a subject developing a careful profile of events and difficulties over the past year. Since many investigators are asking a number of research questions with life events and difficulties representing but one area of interest, some economies often must be made. Our own group is attempting a marriage between the *Dohrenwend* and *Brown* approaches. We are hoping that the PERI, which is more time efficient, will still, if augmented by suitable interviewer probes, yield a relatively complete events picture. At the same time, we are retaining *Brown's* contextual ratings to help reduce error variance which results from including trivial events or events which should more appropriately be viewed as symptoms or products of illness or psychopathology. This strategy should also allow us to determine whether scores derived from ratings by subjects (which is what the PERI requires) are as good at predicting health change as contextual scores derived from *Brown and Harris* [1978].

Social Supports: Independent or Moderator Variable

A number of investigators have suggested that some of the low prediction of symptoms from life events comes from failure of many studies to consider a person's social context. Several models relating events, social supports, and health change have been proposed [see *Dohrenwend and Dohrenwend,* 1984, for a discussion], but for our purposes only two need be considered. The first of these is that social supports (or, more specifically, an inadequate or impoverished social support system) will contribute directly and independently to adverse health. In effect, it could be argued that extreme isolation, loneliness, boredom and friendlessness can be stressors in their own right. The nature of social supports might, under some circumstances, actually condition the occurrence of undesirable events. For example, an occurrence such as bankruptcy, unquestionably a highly threatening event, might be prevented for a small businessman who has good social supports but unavoidable for one who is weak in these. If social supports are construed as an independent variable contributing to health change, then their role in the context of stressful events can be either additive or interactive. An additive phenomenon would exist if both life events and social supports independently produced adverse health effects and if the amount of health impact from each source was not affected by the amount of the other influence which was present. An interactive model would operate if both life events and inadequate social supports each produced a health impact in their own right, *and* that impact was markedly heightened when both influences were present simultaneously.

The second major model for implicating social supports in health change is the moderator or stress-buffering role [*Gore,* 1984]. Those who subscribe to this model generally believe that high social supports can markedly attenuate the impact of threatening events, that inadequate social supports can heighten their health impact, but that those social supports in and of themselves (in the absence of a threatening event) have no major health impact. Put in statistical terms, a two-way analysis of variance with life events and social supports entered as independent factors and health status as dependent, this model would produce a main effect for events, no effect for social supports, and an interaction between supports and events. The first model would have produced a main effect *both* for events and social supports, with or without an interaction.

At the present state of our knowledge it is not possible to say which of these two principal models of the role of social supports and health change will be proved correct. Beyond the fact that there has not been a large number of studies, is the thorny issue of how social support is to be measured and analyzed. Some have favored using rather narrow constructs (e.g. isolation), whilst others have used more broad categories such as instrumental support and emotional support. There are problems both ways. In the first instance, an overly restrictive definition might miss important aspects of the meaning of social support; at the other extreme, an overly broad definition might simply measure general life satisfaction, which in itself might be strongly related to the health outcome which is being predicted [readers wishing to pursue the issue of social support further can consult *Cobb, 1976; Dean and Lin, 1977; Eaton, 1978; Gore, 1984; Lin* et al., *1979*].

Personal Characteristics and the Environment – Health Relationship

Even if events, difficulties, and poor social supports can be demonstrated to affect health, this action occurs at an individual level, which means that certain personal characteristics can be expected to play a role in whether adverse social environment does, in fact, proceed to illness. Many personal characteristics might potentially be of importance, but two key variables must be preexisting state of health and nature of the individual's coping skills. Thus, in the case of a neurological illness such as multiple sclerosis, it might plausibly be argued that someone who already is symptomatic is more likely to develop more symptoms in the context of environmental stress than a patient whose disease is completely quiescent. Beyond this, individuals who do not have any neurological disease should be least likely to develop neurological symptoms in relation to stress.

The role of the second personal factor, coping, is more difficult to determine. Coping is difficult to define, although most investigators would agree that it describes efforts to manage the internal and external effects of life circumstances. The literature on coping and adaptation is vast and ranges from psychoanalytic notions of ego adaptive mechanisms to more cognitive-psychological constructs. Unfortunately, research into the relationship of coping to the stress-strain transaction is still in its infancy. *Lazarus* and associates have suggested that coping repertoires can be grouped as 'problem focused' (direct action) and 'emotion focused' (palliation) [*Lazarus and Launier,* 1978]. Although there is some preliminary evidence that problem-focused coping is associated with less psychiatric symptomatology [*Folkman and Lazarus,* 1980], the issue is complex. For example, denial can be thought of as an emotion-focused coping strategy. Under some circumstances persons who deny have more favorable health outcomes. For example, *Stern* et al. [1976] found that patients with myocardial infarction showed less symptoms and a generally better outcome if they tended to cope with denial and optimism during their acute illness. On the other hand, denial has been seen to relate to increased episodes of hospitalizations in patients with asthma [*Staudenmayer* et al., 1979]. In this study, persons who coped with the opposite of denial, i.e. hypervigilance, tended to self-medicate earlier and take other precautionary measures that avoided evolution of a full blown asthmatic attack requiring medical care.

In summary, research on the relationship of the social environment to health has grown steadily and has produced improved methodology and better theoretical models with which to understand the stress-strain relationship. In the section which follows, some of the applications of this type of research to neurological disease will be considered.

The Epileptogenicity of Psychosocial Factors

Epilepsy has been defined as a paroxysmal and transitory disturbance of the functions of the brain which develops suddenly, ceases spontaneously, and exhibits a conspicuous tendency to recurrence [*Brain and Walton,* 1969]. Historically, efforts to understand epilepsy have been intimately interwined with the history of psychopathology. Until the beginning of the 20th century epilepsy was commonly thought to be caused or provoked by external influences such as divine intervention, possession by evil spirits, or the result of moral turpitude [*Blumer and Benson,* 1982]. With the growth of neurology and neuropathology as clinical sciences in the late 1900s, and, particularly, with the discovery of effective anticonvulsants in the first half of the 20th century, the pendulum has swung to the extent that many clinicians believe that psychosocial factors have little relevance in the understanding of epilepsy. For example, *Brain's Diseases of the Nervous System* states: 'these (psychological factors) are relatively unimportant. It is doubtful if psychological factors alone are sufficient to cause epileptic convulsions. In individuals otherwise predisposed, however, fright or anxiety may precipitate attacks' [*Brain and Walton,* 1969, p. 922]. On the other hand, *Laidlaw and Richens* [1976] in their textbook of epilepsy comment 'many patients and their physicians believe that emotional stress can favor the occurrence of fits and there is evidence for a clinical group where seizures occur only after stress' (p. 457).

There are two principal reasons for a divergence of opinion on the potential epileptogenicity of psychosocial factors. The first is that vague terms such as 'emotional stress' and 'psychological factors' are often used without acknowledgment of the multifactorial nature of the social environment and the difficulties inherent in measuring them (see discussion of this in the first part of the chapter); the second problem has been the dearth of studies which are methodologically sound – rather, opinion has tended to predominate where scientific evidence simply does not exist. Nevertheless, it is important to have some familiarity with what has been observed, as this can form the basis for more satisfactory research efforts in the future.

Affect and Seizures

Although there are many anecdotal statements to the effect that fear, rage and other powerful affects can trigger fits, *Gastaut and Tassinari* [1966] were not able to uncover definitive evidence that such induction occurs. In the laboratory, with EEG monitoring, some epileptics who are rendered emotionally tense and apprehensive show stress-induced augmentation of the photomyocolonic flicker response [*Alter and Hauser,* 1972]. However, such myogenic frontal spiking is not accompanied by authentic cerebral spikes or spike wave complexes, i.e. the photomyocolonic response should be not confused with the protoconvulsive response.

On the other hand, some workers using EEG monitoring and, in one instance, even videotape monitoring of epileptics have produced preliminary evidence that affective changes can produce abnormal EEG patterns in susceptible patients. For example, *Stevens* [1959] showed that emotionally stressful interviews produced EEG abnormalities in many of her epileptic patients. Similar findings were reported by *Berkhout* et al. [1969].

Stores and Lwin [1981] used continuous Medilog recording of the EEG and diaries by parents, teachers or nurses to monitor the relationship of seizure activity to psychological or psychosocial factors in 28 children aged 6–16. In 5 of these children, the authors were able to establish a relationship between factors such as worry, boredom, drowsiness, physical activity, and hunger and epileptic discharge.

Feldman and Paul [1976] point out that one rate-limiting step in efforts to find associations between emotional triggers and fits using interview methods with patients has to do with the fact that a period of retrograde amnesia frequently accompanies a convulsion. This can mean that potentially important triggering events are erased from the patient's memory. To explore this possibility, these authors examined 5 patients with long-standing complex symptomatology whose fits were thought by patient and physician to be induced by psychosocial stress, but where definitive evidence as to the nature of these emotional triggers was missing. Patients were asked to listen to tape recordings which contained conversations involving various kinds of interpersonal conflict of varying intensity. For each of these patients it was possible to confront them with a conflictual situation which succeeded in producing an epileptic discharge. Patients were unable to recall the details of the trigger situations, but, since the sessions were videotaped, the investigators were able on subsequent occasions to demonstrate to patients how they responded and the specific stimuli which they found stressful. This type of revelation, which was designed to circumvent the peri-ictal amnesia, was thought by the investigators to be helpful in teaching patients cognitive techniques of subsequent avoidance of situations which were epileptogenic for them.

Chronic Life Stress and Seizures

There have been no systematic studies involving the sorts of life events methodology described previously to look into the relationship between acute or chronic life stress and frequency of fits. Several groups of investigators have commented that higher levels of sustained stress are associated with increased seizure activity [*Currie* et al., 1971; *Friis and Lund,* 1974; *Mattson* et al., 1974]. *Aird* [1983], who examined seizure-inducing factors in 500 drug-resistant patients, commented that intense emotional reactions were the most common inducing factors in his study group, although he felt these were not always the 'most important'. He noted also that chronic stress responses were often complicated by other known epileptogenic influences, e.g. excessive use of alcohol and sleep deprivation. Nevertheless, he was able to demonstrate in a case study in which none of the complicating factors was operating, that removal of a patient from a chronically stressful home environment resulted in virtually complete amelioration of her previously anti-convulsant resistant epilepsy.

Sleep deprivation is one of the best established of the epileptogenic factors, being, in fact, a diagnostically employed stressor in the electrophysiological evaluation of many patients. As indicated above, sleep deprivation may be an important factor in its own right, and might be a complicating feature of conditions which produce chronic emotional arousal, e.g. chronic anxiety and chronic depression.

One of the most persuasive demonstrations of the epileptogenic potential of sleep deprivation was by *Gunderson* et al. [1973] who reported on the incidence of seizures in US servicemen returning to California from Vietnam. Most of these servicemen ended up being sleep deprived for periods of 24–48 h as the result of a combination of factors: round-the-clock 'partying' to celebrate their imminent departure from the combat zone; lengthy processing both in Vietnam and in California in anticipation of their discharge; and a long uncomfortable flight across the Pacific which spanned many time zones and afforded little opportunity for continuous sleep. The authors found that the incidence of seizures (in men not previously known to be epileptic) was several hundred times higher than that expected in a non-sleep-deprived civilian population of comparable age. The attack rate increased as function of length of sleep deprivation, with the highest incidence being in those deprived for 37 h or more.

Cognitive Factors and Seizures

A number of perceptual epileptogenic triggers have long been recognized. These stimuli, which can include visual patterns, musical sounds, startle, and reading have been associated with what is termed 'pattern epilepsy'.

More recently investigators have examined cognitive events which by nature of their inherent difficulty or frustration-induction might increase the number of fits in vulnerable individuals. Laboratory studies involving telemetered EEG have led to the observation that ordinary intellectual work which did not place excessive or unaccustomed demands on the patient was not related to EEG abnormalities; on the other hand, problems which exceeded a patient's capacity to solve them tended to increase electrical abnormality [*Vidart and Geier*, 1978; *Bureau* et al., 1968]. *Forster* et al. [1975] reported on a patient who had seizures while playing chess or cards, doing complicated mathematical problems, or during neuropsychological testing. They reviewed a report from China by *Ch'en* et al. [1965] which reported 4 cases of patients experiencing seizures while playing chess or cards.

While cognitive stress might produce EEG abnormalities conducive to increased seizure activity, this does not mean that absence of cognitive activity is necessarily salutary. For example, *Lubar* [1978] noted that techniques of relaxation which did not maintain a mental focus sometimes heightened seizure activity.

Some Potential Physiological Mediators

While it is clear that there are at least some individuals who become susceptible to increased seizure activity as a result of emotional or cognitive factors, the mechanism of this link remains obscure. *Mattson* et al. [1970] suggested that emotional arousal is accompanied by hyperventilation, which produces a physiological state that lowers seizure threshold. Sleep disturbance often accompanies periods of psychological distress, and may be a second factor. In children and adolescents, periods of emotional upheaval may be accompanied by disturbances in feeding. Resultant periods of relative hypoglycemia might be further triggers to increased epilepsy. Finally, both affective and cognitive events are accompanied by complex changes in central neurohumors. As of this writing, no associations have yet been uncovered between changes in monoaminergic-cholinergic balance, GABA, peptide neurotransmitters, and the emotional triggers that have been described, although some interactions are further speculated on in the chapter by *Trimble* (p. 133). The next phase of research into psychosocial factors in epilepsy must approach these neurochemical events on the one hand, and relate them to more sophisticated measures of patients' life circumstances, on the other. In the meantime, the model for the relationship between stress, epilepsy, and sleep proposed by *Trimble and Wilson-Barnett* [1982] seems serviceable, and can be used as a departure point for further research (fig. 1).

Psychosocial Factors in Stroke

Strokes consist of catastrophic interruptions of cerebral oxygenation occasioned by thromboembolic events or hemorrhages into the brain or subarachnoid space.

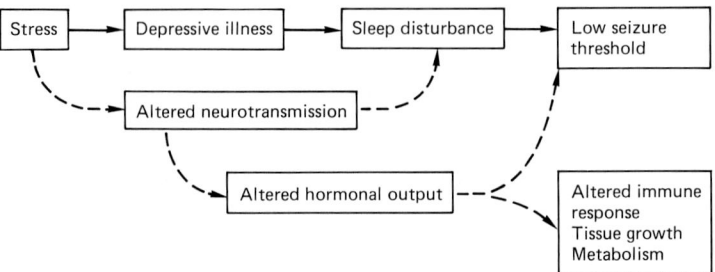

Fig. 1. Relationships between stress and seizures.

The very term 'stroke' is laden with emotional meanings, and one can find references throughout the recorded history of medicine to the effect that strokes can be caused by severe emotional upset. Even now we say things like 'don't say that to him – he'll have a stroke!'.

According to *Adler* et al. [1971], *Johann Wepfer* first commented, in 1658, on 2 cases of apoplexy preceded by emotional upheaval. One of his patients was Malpighi who 'was seized, in the sixty-sixth year of his age with an apoplexy, ushered in with care, passions of the mind, etc.' [*Adler* et al., 1971, p. 2]. 200 years later, *Tuke* [1982], in his 'Influences of the mind on the body' reported that a 56-year-old woman suffered a cerebral hemorrhage shortly after being threatened with violence.

Benjamin Rush, America's first psychiatrist, reported that there was an increase in apoplexy in Philadelphia during the years 1774–1775, immediately preceding the Declaration of Independence which was 'a period of uncommon anxiety among the citizens of America' [*Adler* et al., 1971, p. 2]. In a similar vein, *Halliday* [1948] demonstrated a rise in the incidence of stroke in Scotland between the years 1931 and 1936, a period of economic depression in that country. The greatest rise was among those under 55 (i.e. in persons who would normally be at lower risk).

More systematic observations into the role of life stress and the emotions in the genesis of stroke took place in the middle of the 20th century, beginning with the work of *Ecker* and associates. In their first report, *Seidenberg and Ecker* [1953] provided detailed case histories on 6 patients who experienced a stroke characterized by some combination of sudden onset of impaired consciousness and hemiparesis. 4 cases involved cerebral hemorrhage and all were thought to have vasospasm involving the internal carotid circulation. Three patients died. Antecedent stressful events were noted in each case; furthermore, the authors believed that each patient had personality disturbances, difficulty in handling hostility and anger, in particular.

In a subsequent report on a larger series of cases, *Ecker* [1954] described 20 cases of stroke, which included 13 cases of nontraumatic intracranial bleeding and 8 of hemiparesis (1 case had both). The author noted antecedent stressful events in virtually all of the cases. Furthermore, 13 of the 20 cases were described as having character pathology involving difficulties in the management of anger and hostility. Vasospasm was demonstrated in 15 angiographed cases. The author suggested that acute and chronic emotional tension, particularly tension related to the management of anger, can lead to vasospasm which then can predispose to stroke.

There were many difficulties with these two studies, both from psychological and medical standpoints. For example, it seemed entirely possible that the contrast medium used (Diodrast) might itself cause spasm. Furthermore, since arteriography was conducted after the stroke, the possibility that pathogenic processes (e.g. presence of blood in the subarachnoid space) might be causing and maintaining spasm could not be excluded. Finally, the method of gathering personality and life events information, and its exact association with the onset of stroke was not established in a convincing fashion. Nevertheless, this set of studies represents the first systematic effort to examine the issue.

The next major report came from *Storey* [1969] whose review of 261 patients with proved subarachnoid hemorrhage revealed several dramatic cases of bleeding after severe emotional shock. For example, 1 woman aged 50 suffered a hemorrhage immediately after a policeman came suddenly to her door and announced that the woman next door, who was her closest friend, had hanged herself in the lavatory. Another woman suffered a subarachnoid hemorrhage 'from within a minute of being told by her husband that he was going to divorce her for adultery – which she thought he knew nothing about' [*Storey*, 1969, p. 177]. Such dramatic associations, albeit uncommon, nevertheless suggest that in certain vulnerable individuals intense emotional upset can precipitate a subarachnoid hemorrhage. *Storey* [1969; chapt. 4] observed further that there was a greater tendency for life events and emotional factors to be salient in patients who experienced subarachnoid bleeds without concomitant evidence of presence of an aneurysm.

The theme that there might be a differential vulnerability to life stress in cases of nonaneurysm intracranial bleeds was picked up by *Penrose* [1972]. He performed a retrospective study with 44 patients who experienced a subarachnoid hemorrhage. Using reports of knowledgable significant others, he conducted a life events interview using an earlier version of the Bedford College instrument described by *Brown and Birley* [1968]. Patients were roughly equally divided into those who did and did not have berry aneurysms. 48% of the nonaneurysm strokes experienced a significant event in the three weeks prior to their stroke; by way of comparison 28% of the berry aneurysm cases and 19% of *Brown and Birley's* controls reported such events. The mechanism of this apparent differential vulnerability is not clear, although the author suggested that greater vasomotor reactivity might be a factor in some patients.

Another report on emotional factors in cerebral vascular disease came from *Adler* et al. [1971]. These investigators performed very detailed psychological analyses (often involving many sessions of psychodynamic psychotherapy) with 32 men who between them experienced 35 strokes. They observed that strokes typically occurred during a period of sustained emotional difficulty. For example, in 27 of the 35 stroke episodes personal failing presented as an important circumstance. In 19 instances difficult environmental demands, burdens, or obstacles 'which blocked activity or thwarted fulfillment' were noted. Events or circumstances related to loss of status, loss of control, and real or threatened object loss were also noted with regularity. From a personality standpoint, *Adler* and associates thought that the stroke patients shared similarities with the typical coronary artery type 'A' personality, and that they also had some of the characteristics which have been ascribed to persons with hypertension – in particular, difficulty in controlling anger, which tends to be consciously suppressed or unconsciously repressed.

From this brief review it can be seen that work on efforts to relate psychosocial influences to cerebrovascular accident is still in its infancy. It seems clear that in a few predisposed individuals catastrophic life events can lead within minutes to an intercranial hemorrhage. It seems possible, also, that chronic stress, punctuated by an exacerbation of life events can lead to increases in blood pressure and/or vasospasm which can predispose to onset of bleeding. A possible model for the relationship between biological and environmental factors in the genesis of stroke is presented in figure 2. This was modified from *Steptoe* [1981] who developed it initially as a model to understand the genesis of hypertension.

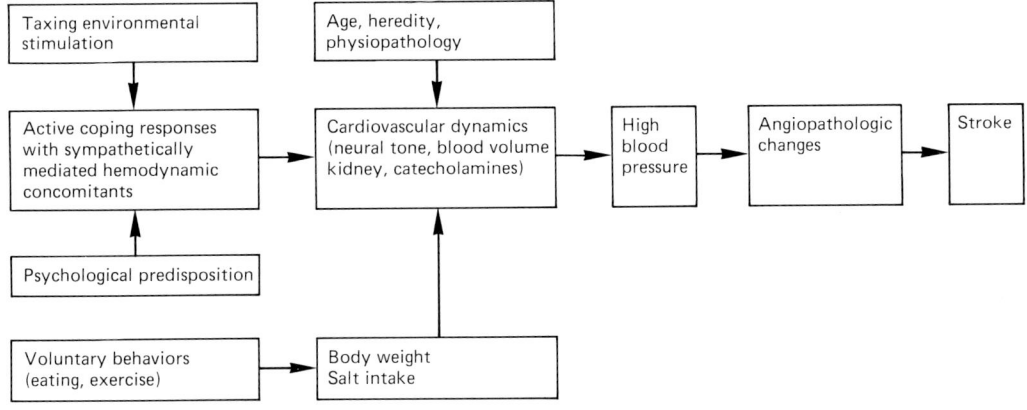

Fig. 2. Behavioral and psychological contributions to stroke.

Psychosocial Influences on the Onset and Exacerbation of Symptoms of Multiple Sclerosis

Of the three neurological entities reviewed here, multiple sclerosis has been studied most extensively from the standpoint that environmental stresses might contribute to the onset or worsening of symptoms. The review by *Warren* et al. [1982] notes that what is probably our earliest description of a case of multiple sclerosis, that of the illness of Augustus d'Este (1782–1846) records that this patient's disease began 'immediately after he attended the funeral of a father figure' [*Warren* et al., 1982, p. 821]. The occasional relationship of emotional shock to onset of symptoms has received comment from many authorities including *Charcot, Bramwell* and *McAlpine,* and is further discussed in chapter 5.

In the middle of the 20th century, several groups of investigators began to look at the role of psychosocial stress in multiple sclerosis in more detail. *Langworthy* and associates described several patients whose symptoms were aggravated when they were caught in an interpersonal situation characterized by being controlled and dominated, with a feeling that they were hopelessly trapped in such a situation [*Langworthy* 1948, 1950; *Langworthy and LeGrand,* 1952].

Brickner and Simons [1950] noted that in 16 of 50 patients whom they studied, emotional stress seemed to be a factor in precipating symptom exacerbation. *Grinker* et al., [1950] also reported that their 26 patients with multiple sclerosis showed development of overt neurological symptomatology in relation to major changes in life circumstances. *Philippopoulos* et al., [1958] agreed that traumatic experiences were important, but emphasized the role of prolonged emotional stress, which they noted in 35 of their 40 patients.

Engel and colleagues performed a detailed psychodynamic study of 32 patients from the United States and Israel who developed multiple sclerosis. They were particularly interested in the transitional period between health and disease. These authors suggested that in 28 of their 32 patients this transition coincided with the occurrence of a psychologically stressful situation, one which mobilized feelings of helplessness [*Mei-Tal* et al., 1970]. This theme of psychological coping being overwhelmed as a precursor to onset of symptoms was echoed by *Groen* et al. [1967].

During the same period several negative results emerged, as well. *Pratt* [1951] compared a group of 100 patients with multiple sclerosis to a similar number with other neurological illnesses. He was unable to find a statistically significant association between life stress or emotional upset and onset or exacerbation of illness (although he did note that patients with multiple sclerosis tended to report more stressful circumstances). Similarly, *Braceland and Giffin* [1950] noted no differences in reports of stressful life events between patients with multiple sclerosis and neurological controls, and *Alter* et al. [1968] found no significant differences between MS patients and nonpatient controls.

Two recent studies have again suggested that stressful life circumstances may be associated with onset or exacerbation of symptoms. *Warren* et al. [1982] performed interviews with 100 patients with multiple sclerosis and 100 control patients with other neurological or musculoskeletal diseases. The authors found that patients with MS experienced three times as many events as controls in the two year period prior to onset. Furthermore, significantly more MS cases than neuromuscular controls reported three or more events in the 2-year time frame. Events included personal illness or illness of a close family member, interactional problems with a family member, marital difficulties, pregnancy-related problems, financial problems, and changes in residence or life style.

Our own group has recently completed a detailed study of life events and difficulties in 40 patients with multiple sclerosis, focusing on the 1-year period preceding onset of major symptomatology [*Grant* et al., in preparation]. We used the method of *Brown and Harris* [1978], which involved a lengthy (approximately 2 h) personal interview between one of the investigators and the patient. The interview attempted to elicit information regarding life happenings in the areas of health of important others, role changes, interaction changes, important news or forecasts, and miscellaneous other life crises for the year preceeding symptom onset. Events were then assigned contextual ratings of severity of threat by the investigators. This allowed partitioning of events by threat level into 'severe' and 'nonsevere' events.

We found that 72% of our MS patients experienced at least one severely threatening event in the year preceding major symptom onset. A comparable rate for nonpatients derived from *Brown and Harris*' community sample was 20%. This is a highly significant difference, and the rate for patients is comparable to that reported by *Brown and Harris* [1978] for the period prior to onset of major depression in their psychiatric study. It is also comparable to the data of *Warren* et al. [1982] who noted that 79% of their patients reported more 'unwanted stress than usual, due to congregation of events'. Despite this superficial similarity with *Warren* et al., because of differences in methodology, it is not clear whether their events would correspond to our category of 'severe threat'.

Thus, at this writing, the role of environmental stressors in the precipitation and exacerbation of symptoms of multiple sclerosis remains unclear. Many older studies, and two recent ones have suggested that there is such a relationship. Several other studies have produced negative results. In any event, none of the recent studies suggests that psychosocial factors contribute aetiologically to multiple sclerosis – rather, these factors can be seen to precipitate or aggravate a biological process that is ongoing. Exactly how psychosocial factors exert their potential role is not clear. We know that severe emotional stress, severe depression in particular, can be associated with changes in immune mechanisms. Since multiple sclerosis is commonly thought to be related at least in part to alterations in the immune system, it is possible to speculate that immune mechanisms which are already compromised can undergo further destabilization under some circumstances in the face of severe or chronic emotional upset. Further progress in this field will occur when careful psychosocial methodology is coupled with equally careful analysis of neuroendocrine and immune status in patients with multiple sclerosis.

Summary

This chapter has reviewed some of the methodological and theoretical issues in research linking the social environment to medical illnesses. The second part of the chapter has focused on three specific neurological entities to examine evidence for a possible association between neurological illness and life stress. There is some suggestion that certain vulnerable epileptic patients can experience convulsions in response to acute emotional upheaval or certain types of cognitive challenges. More commonly, it is probable that social stress and emotional tension can produce lowering of seizure threshold by increasing levels of fatigue and disrupting sleep. The latter factor, in particular, is known to lower seizure threshold. In the case of stroke, several dramatic cases of intracranial hemorrhage have been related to disastrous life circumstances. A general association between life stress and stroke has yet to be established. The case for a link between life events and onset of exacerbation of multiple sclerosis seems stronger. Events which produce emotional upset seem capable of worsening symptoms in patients with existing disease, and several studies have reported unusual life stresses in the period preceding onset of symptoms in this disorder.

References

Adler, R.; MacRitchie, K.; Engel, G.L.: Psychologic processes and ischemic stroke (occlusive cerebrovascular disease). Psychosom. Med. *33:* 1–29 (1971).

Alter, M.; Antonovsky, A.; Leibowitz, V.: Epidemiology of multiple sclerosis in Israel; In Alter, Kurtzke, The epidemiology of multiple sclerosis, pp. 83–109 (Thomas, Springfield 1968).

Alter, M.; Hauser, W.A.: The epidemiology of epilepsy. A workshop. NINDS monogr. No. 14 (1972).

Aird, R.B.: The importance of seizure-inducing factors in the control of refractory forms of epilepsy. Epilepsia *24:* 567–582 (1983).

Bennet, G.: Bristol floods, 1968: controlled survey of effect on health of local community disaster. Br. med J. *iii:* 454–458 (1970).

Berkhout, J.; Walter, D.O.; Adey, W.R.: Alterations of the human electroencephalogram induced by stressful verbal activity. Electroenceph. clin. Neurophysiol. *27:* 457–469 (1969).

Blumer, D.; Benson, D.F.: Psychiatric manifestations of epilepsy; in Benson, Blumer, Psychiatric aspects of neurologic disease, No. 2, pp. 25–48 (Grune & Stratton, New York 1982).

Braceland, F.J.; Giffin, M.E.: The mental changes associated with multiple sclerosis. Proc. Ass. Res. nerv. ment. Dis. *28:* 450–455 (1950).

Brain, W.R.; Walton, J.N.: Brain's diseases of the nervous system (Oxford University Press, London 1969).

Brickner, R.; Simons, B.: Emotional stress in relation to attacks of multiple sclerosis. Proc. Ass. Res. nerv. ment. Dis. *28:* 143 (1950).

Brown, G.W.: Contextual measures of life events; in Dohrenwend, Dohrenwend, Stressful life events and their contexts. Series in psychosocial epidemiology, No. 2, pp. 187–201 (Rutgers University Press, New Brunswick 1984).

Brown, G.W.: Meaning, measurement and stress of life events; in Dohrenwend, Dohrenwend, Stressful life events: their nature and effects, pp. 217–243 (Wiley, New York 1974).

Brown, G.W.; Birley, J.L.T.: Crisis and life changes and the onset of schizophrenia. J. Hlth soc. Behav. *9:* 203 (1968).

Brown, G.W.; Harris, T.: Social origins of depression: a study of psychiatric disorder in women (Tavistock, London 1978).

Bureau, et al., 1968: Cited in Laidlaw and Richens: A textbook of epilepsy, p. 256 (Churchill-Livingstone, Edinburgh 1976).

Ch'en, H.P.; Ch'in, D.; Ch'u, C.P.: Chess epilepsy and card epilepsy. Chin. med. J. *84:* 470–474 (1965).

Clayton, P.J.: The sequelae and nonsequelae of conjugal bereavement. Am. J. Psychiat. *136:* 1530–1534 (1979).

Currie, S.; Heathfield, K.W.G.; Henson, R.A.; Scott, D.F.: Clinical course and prognosis of temporal lobe epilepsy. A survey of 666 patients. Brain *94:* 173–190 (1971).

Cobb, S.: Social support as a moderator of life stress. Psychosom. Med. *38:* 300–314 (1976).

Dean, A.; Lin, N.: The stress-buffering role of social support: problems and prospects for systematic investigation. J. nerv. ment. Dis. *165:* 7–15 (1977).

Dohrenwend, B.S.; Dohrenwend, B.P.: Life stress and illness: formulation of the issues; in Dohrenwend, Dohrenwend, Stressful life events and their contexts. Series in psychosocial epidemiology, No. 2, pp. 1–27 (Rutgers University Press, New Brunswick 1984).

Dohrenwend, B.P.; Dohrenwend, B.S.: The conceptualization and measurement of stressful life events: an overview of the issues; in Strauss, Babigian, Roff, The origins and course of psychopathology, pp. 93–116 (Plenum Press, New York 1977).

Dohrenwend, B.S.; Krasnoff, L.; Askenasy, A.R.; Dohrenwend, B.P.: Exemplification of a method for scaling life events. J. Hlth soc. Behav. *19:* 205–229 (1978).

Eaton, W.: Life events, social supports and psychiatric symptoms. A reanalysis of the New Haven data. J. Hlth soc. Behav. *19:* 230–234 (1978).

Ecker, A.: Emotional stress before strokes: a preliminary report of 20 cases. Ann. intern. Med. *40:* 49–56 (1954).

Feldman, R.G.; Paul, N.L.: Identity of emotional triggers in epilepsy. J. nerv. ment. Dis. *162:* 345–353 (1976).

Figley, C.: Stress disorders among Vietnam veterans, theory research and treatment (Brunner/Mazel, New York 1978).

Folkman, S.; Lazarus, R.S.: An analysis of coping in a middle-aged community sample. J. Hlth soc. Behav. *21:* 219–239 (1980).

Forster, F.M.; Richards, J.F.; Panitch, H.S.; Huisman, R.E.; Paulsen, R.E.: Reflex epilepsy evoked by decision making. Archs Neurol. *32:* 54–56 (1975).

Friis, M.L.; Lund, M.: Stress convulsions. Archs Neurol. *31:* 155–159 (1974).

Gastaut, H.; Tassinari, G.A.: Triggering mechanisms in epilepsy. The electroclinical point of view. Epilepsia 7: 85–138 (1968).

Gore, S.: Stress-buffering functions of social supports: an appraisal and clarification of research models; in Dohrenwend, Dohrenwend, Stressful life events and their contexts. Series in psychosocial epidemiology, No. 2, pp. 201–222 (Rutgers University Press, New Brunswick 1984).

Gore, S.: The effect of social support in moderating the health consequences of unemployment. J. Hlth Soc. Behav. 19: 157–165 (1978).

Grant, I.; Sweetwood, H.; Yager, J.; Gerst, M.: Quality of life events in relation to psychiatric symptoms. Archs Gen. Psychiat. 38: 335–339 (1981).

Grant, I.; Yager, J.; Sweetwood, H.; Olshen, R.: Life events and symptoms. Fourier analysis of time series from a three year prospective study. Archs gen. Psychiat. 39: 598–605 (1982).

Grinker, R.; Ham, G.; Robbins, F.: Some psychodynamic factors in multiple sclerosis. Proc. Ass. Res. nerv. ment, Dis. 28: 456 (1950).

Groen, J.J.; Prick, J.J.G.; Bastiaans, J.: Multiple sclerose (De Erven F. Bohn, NV, Haarlem 1967).

Gunderson, C.H.; Dunne, P.B.; Feyer, T.L.: Sleep deprivation seizures. Neurology, Minneap. 23: 678–686 (1973).

Halliday, J.L.: Psychosocial medicine, a study of the sick society (Norton, New York 1948).

Hinkle, L.E.: The effect of exposure to culture change, social change, and changes in interpersonal relationships on health; in Dohrenwend, Dohrenwend, Stressful life events, their nature and effects, pp. 9–44 (Wiley, New York 1974).

Hirschfeld, R.M.A.; Klerman, G.L.; Schless, A.P.; et al.: Modified life events section of the Psychiatric Epidemiology Research Interview (PERI) for use in the clinical studies of the NIMH clinical research branch collaborative program on the psychobiology of depression (1977) (copy supplied by Dr. Hirschfeld).

Holmes, T.H.; Rahe, R.H.: The social readjustment rating scale. J. psychosom. Res. 11: 213–218 (1967).

Kanner, A.D.; Coyne, J.C.; Schaefer, C.; Lazarus, R.S.: Comparison of two modes of stress measurement: daily hassles and uplits versus major life events. J. behav. Med. 4: 1–39 (1981).

Laidlaw, L.; Richens, A.: A textbook of epilepsy (Churchill-Livingstone, Edinburgh 1976).

Langworthy, O.R.: Relation of personality problems to onset and progress of multiple sclerosis. Archs Neurol. Psychiat. 59: 13 (1948).

Langworthy, O.R.; LeGrand, D.: Personality structure and psychotherapy in multiple sclerosis. Am. J. Med. 12: 586 (1952).

Lazarus, R.S.: The costs and benefits of denial; in Dohrenwend, Dohrenwend, Stressful life events and their contexts. Series in psychosocial epidemiology, No. 2, pp. 131–156 (Rutgers University Press, New Brunswick 1984).

Lazarus, R.S.; Launier, R.: Stress-related transactions between person and environment; in Pervin, Lewis, Perspectives in interactional psychology, pp. 287–327 (Plenum Press, New York 1978).

Lin, N.; Simeone, R.S.; Ensel, W.; Kuo, W.: Social support, stressful life events and illness: a model and empirical test. J. Hlth soc. Behav. 20: 108–119 (1979).

Lubar, J.G.: Clinical applications of EEG feedback, including treatment of epilepsy. Biomedical Services, Inc., Clinical Biofeedback Seminar, San Francisco 1978.

Masuda, M.; Holmes, T.H.: Magnitude estimations of social readjustments. J. psychosom. Res. *11:* 219–225 (1967).

Mattson, R.; Lerner, E.; Dix, G.: Precipitating and inhibiting factors in epilepsy: a statistical study. Epilepsia *15:* 271–272 (1974).

Mei-Tal, V.; Meyerowitz, S.; Engel, G.L.: The role of psychological process in a somatic disorder: multiple sclerosis. Psychosom. Med. *32:* 67–86 (1970).

Monroe, S.M.: Major and minor life events as predictors of psychological distress: further issues and findings. J. behav. Med. *6:* 189–205 (1983).

Monroe, S.; Imhoff, D.F.; Wise, B.D.; Harris, J.E.: Prediction of psychological symptoms under high-risk psychosocial circumstances: life events, social support and symptom specificity. J. abnorm. Psychol. *92:* 338–350 (1983).

Parkes, C.M.; Benjamin, B.; Fitzgerald, R.G.: Broken heart. A statistical study of increased mortality among widowers. Br. med. J. *i:* 740–743 (1969).

Paykel, E.; Myers, J.; Dienelt, M.N.; Klerman, J.; Lindenthal, J.; Pepper, M.: Life events and depression: a controlled study. Archs gen. Psychiat. *21:* 753–760 (1969).

Penrose, R.J.J.: Life events before subarachnoid haemorrhage. J. psychosom. Res. *16:* 329–333 (1972).

Philippopoulos, G.S.; Wittkower, E.D.; Cousineau, A.: The etiologic significance of emotional factors in onset and exacerbations of multiple sclerosis. Psychosom. Med. *20:* 458–474 (1958).

Pratt, R.T.C.: An investigation of the psychiatric aspects of disseminated sclerosis. J. Neurol. Neurosurg. Psychiat. *14:* 326–336 (1951).

Rabkin, J.G.; Struening, E.L.: Life events, stress and illness. Science *194:* 1013–1020 (1976).

Rahe, R.H.: In Gunderson, Rahe, Life change and subsequent illness reports, pp. 58–78 (Thomas, Springfield 1974).

Rahe, R.H.; Arthur, R.J.: Life change and illness studies: past history and future directions. J. human. Stress *4:* 3–15 (1978).

Rahe, R.H.; Meyer, M.; Smith, M.; Kjaer, G.; Holmes, T.H.: Social stress and illness onset. J. psychosom. Res. *8:* 35–44 (1964).

Seidenberg, R.; Ecker, A.: Psychodynamic and arteriographic studies of acute cerebral vascular disorders. Psychosom. Med. *16:* 374–392 (1953).

Staudenmayer, H.; Kinsman, R.A.; Dirk, J.F.; Spector, S.L.; Wangaard, C.: Medical outcome in asthmatic patients. Effects of airways hyperactivity and symptom-focused anxiety. Psychosom. Med. *41:* 109–118 (1979).

Steptoe, A.: Psychological factors in cardiovascular disorders, p. 153 (Academic Press, London 1981).

Stern, M.J.; Pascale, L.; McLoone, J.B.: Psychosocial adaptation following an acute myocardial infarction. J. chron. Dis. *29:* 313–526 (1976).

Stevens, J.R.: Emotional activation of the electroencephalogram in patients with convulsive disorders. J. nerv. ment. Dis. *128:* 339–351 (1959).

Stores, G.; Lwin, R.: In Dam, Gram, Penry, A study of factors associated with the occurrence of generalized seizure discharge in children with epilepsy using the Oxford Medilog system for ambulatory monitoring, pp. 421–422 (Raven Press, New York 1981).

Storey, P.B.: The precipitation of subarachnoid haemorrhage. J. psychosom. Res. *13:* 175–182 (1969).

Swinyard, E.A.; Clark, L.D.; Miyahara, J.T.; Wolf, H.H.: Studies on the mechanism of amphetamine toxicity in aggregated mice. J. Pharmac. exp. Ther. *132:* 97–102 (1961).

Swinyard, E.A.; Miyahara, J.T.; Clark, L.D.; Goodman, L.S.: The effect of experimentally induced stress on pentylenetetrazol seizure threshold in mice. Psychopharmacologia *4:* 343–353 (1963).

Swinyard, E.A.; Radhakrishnan, N.; Goodman, L.S.: Effect of brief restraint on the convulsive threshold of mice. J. Pharmac. exp. Ther. *38:* 337–342 (1962).

Trimble, M.R.; Wilson-Barnett, J.: Neuropsychiatric aspects of stress. Practitioner *226:* 1580–1586 (1982).

Tuke, D.H.: Influence of the mind upon the body, p. 264 (Lindsay & Blakeston, Philadelphia 1872).

Vidart, L.; Geier, S.: Minor epileptic attacks: description and electroclinical correlation. Electroenceph. clin. Neurophysiol. *30:* 371 (1971).

Warren, S.; Greenhill, S.; Warren, K.G.: Emotional stress and the development of multiple sclerosis. Case-control evidence of a relationship. J. chron. Dis. *35:* 821–831 (1982).

Yager, J.; Grant, I.; Sweetwood, H.; Gerst, M.S.: Life event reports by psychiatric patients, nonpatients and their partners. Archs gen. Psychiat. *38:* 343–347 (1981).

Dr. Igor Grant, Psychiatry Service (116), VA Medical Center,
3350 La Jolla Village Drive, San Diego, CA 92161 (USA)

3. Head Injury, Neurosis and Accident Proneness

A.C.P. Sims

Department of Psychiatry, St. James's University Hospital, Leeds, UK

Case Report

Miss A., age 20 years, received a head injury in a road accident in Italy. She was admitted to hospital in Italy, transferred to an accident ward in England, and later to a psychiatric hospital.

Her father was a kind, well-meaning man of strict morals and high standards. Miss A. described her mother as 'volatile, extravagant, and needing attention'. The patient was an only child in a family without psychiatric history, but with severe marital conflict; her parents separated and reunited several times with eventual divorce.

Miss A. lived with her mother. At the age of 8 she was put on probation for shop-lifting; at 11 she passed examination to grammar school; at 13 her mother became considerably in debt and when creditors visited the house Miss A. was sent to dismiss them with lies. At this time she developed a complete inability to walk and was admitted to hospital; she was seen by a psychiatrist after organic illness had been excluded. Complete recovery occurred and she remained well until the age of 16 years. She then developed amenorrhoea and anorexia lasting for 6 months, which ended when her father, at his home, refused to let her out of the house until she reached what he considered a satisfactory weight. At the age of 18 she gained four good 'A' level passes and a place at university to read psychology. She completed 2 years at university with examination results suggesting an eventual upper second class degree. According to her father, she had always tended to be shallow, exuberant, and transitory in her relationships and, more recently, promiscuous. He also described her dishonesty, and her similarity to her mother in her flamboyant and extravagant nature. She had, in her flat, for instance, 5 pairs of boots almost unworn, large numbers of books, many of them duplicate copies, and piles of notepads and boxes of pens, mostly new. He suspected that some of these had been stolen, and indeed she had received a conditional discharge for stealing a pair of sunglasses before going on holiday.

A friend described her as 'trying to get too much of the limelight' which was beginning to annoy others. Miss A. described herself as deeply interested in psychology and as 'extroverted'.

Table I. Serial intellectual assessment (using WAIS) after head injury

Test results	Number of days after head injury			
	12	26	53	222
Full scale WAIS	test abandoned	92	117	120
Verbal		97	116	119
Performance		87	115	119

Present Illness

In her vacation she had hitch-hiked with a friend. Reckless driving had ended with Miss A.'s ejection from the car with a resultant closed head injury and concussion. She had been admitted to hospital and, on recovery of consciousness, 'talked rubbish', was disorientated in time and space, and was drowsy.

On her return to the United Kingdom, her conversation was found to be indistinct, repetitive, slow, and at times nonsensical. She was drowsy and slept for large parts of the day. Skull X-ray and neurological examination were normal. She then became flirtatious with all men, and 'a nuisance' to the nursing staff. Psychiatric referral followed, and her mental state was normal, except for frivolity and amorousness with the giving of approximate answers, thus: Q: 'What is the capital of Italy?' – A: 'Naples'; Q: 'What is the capital of Scotland?' – A: 'Aberdeen'; Q: 'How many legs has a centipede?' – A: '7'. She also showed emotional lability and a period of total amnesia. She did not show perseveration.

2 weeks after the accident on transfer to psychiatric hospital, approximate answers were usually accompanied by explanations or expletives, and accurate answers by nothing, thus: Q: '14+15?' – A:'37 – oh, I'm sorry'; Q: '9+8?' – A: '17'; Q: '4×13?' – A: '53 – jeepers, I've never been very good at arithmetic'; Q: 'Capital of Spain?' – A: 'Dunno'; Q: 'Capital of Japan?' – A: 'Tokyo'; Q: 'Capital of Scotland?' – A: 'Blimey, Aberdeen'; Q: 'How many of each suit in a pack of cards? – A: '14 ... 13, sorry, my maths is bad, ... 13 ... 14, jeepers creepers'.

With the test of serial sevens she counted on her fingers and made occasional small mistakes. This was accompanied by 'its not an attention-getting thing – I'm just trying to answer your questions'.

Questions directed towards orientation were answered with varying degrees of accuracy, thus: 'Where are you?' 'The nerve part of the hospital'.

During the lengthy interview she at no time expressed surprise at such questions as 'how many legs has a centipede?', and did not contradict herself. She dissolved in tears with anxiety about her ability to continue her course at one moment, and was flirting with the examiner the next. There was no evidence at any time of hallucinations or delusions.

Physical examination was normal, apart from a healing laceration, as were clinical investigations. The results of serial psychological testing are summarised in table I. There was an initial discrepancy between verbal and performance scores as expected with organic damage. This was seen to resolve with a steady improvement in Full Scale Score, which did not, however, reach the standard expected of an above-average psychology student.

During her stay in hospital (day 11 to day 59 after the accident) Miss A. interfered with the treatment of other patients, played staff off against patients and vice versa, and made frank declarations of love to one of the medical staff in daily lengthy letters, written more in the style of a young schoolgirl than an intelligent student. However, without medication or other specific treatment, her mental state improved in parallel with her WAIS test. She became fully orientated, and her amorous approaches became less blatant. In out-patient follow-up, she showed a continued improvement in psychometric testing, and she returned to university. Even 5 months after the accident she still gave approximate answers, thus: 'How many legs has a centipede?' – '16', and 'What is the capital of Italy?' – 'Naples'. However, 7 months after the accident she gave no such answers and had gained the highest mark in her university course for an essay.

Her comparatively poor final WAIS results could be explained by a certain residual flippancy towards such tests. It was felt by her father that she had returned to her normal self, both in terms of intellect and personality. She expressed surprise at having answered questions as she had done, and claimed to have no memory for her approximations [*Latcham* et al., 1978].

This case demonstrates very clearly the complicated relationship between head injury, neurosis and *pre-morbid personality*. She gave *approximate answers*, showed *clouding of consciousness*, had experienced head injury, manifested *'hysterical'* stigmata, and had experienced *amnesia* for the period during which these symptoms were manifest; these are positive features for the psychopathology of *Ganser syndrome* [*Ganser*, 1898]. She did not show hallucinations nor was she a criminal; although these features appeared in *Ganser's* original description they are not required for diagnosis of the syndrome [*Curran and Partridge*, 1969; *Enoch and Irving*, 1962; *Whitlock*, 1967; *Tsoi*, 1973].

The patient had a clear previous diagnosis of *hysterical neurosis*, and a *premorbid* personality of *hysterical* type. She was consistently attention-seeking and histrionic in her behaviour. She also had a severe head injury with prolonged alteration of consciousness. She had already formed neurotic patterns of behaviour, both in terms of isolated episodes of conversion hysteria and consistent personality traits, before her head injury. It is not then surprising that added to her organic brain symptoms were also reactive symptoms to the distress, and fear engendered in coping with her injury and its potential consequences.

The Psychosomatic Conundrum: Brain and Behaviour

Lipowski [1976] has defined psychosomatic medicine as follows: '(1) *A science* of the *relationships* between psychological, biological and social variables as they pertain to human health and disease; (2) *an approach* to the *practice* of medicine that advocates the inclusion of psychosocial factors in the study, prevention, diagnosis and management of all diseases; (3) *clinical activities* at the interface of medicine and behavioural sciences subsumed under the term "consultation-liaison psychiatry".'

At its most inclusive, therefore, it incorporates almost every medical condition; when used in too narrow a sense it makes assumptions about aetiology which are not justified by evidence. *Granville-Grossman* [1983] has listed the different relationships between mind and body in physical and psychiatric disorder: '(1) Some physical illness may be psychogenic, i.e. the mental disturbance is a cause of the physical illness. (2) Physical illness may arise as an indirect consequence of the mental disorder, the bodily illness resulting from behavioural disturbances secondary to the psychiatric abnormality. (3) Physical methods of treatment of psychiatric illness may sometimes cause somatic disease. (4) The mental disorder may be an organically determined manifestation of the physical illness or an adverse effect of its treatment. (5) The psychiatric disturbance may represent a psychological reaction to the significance of the physical illness and of its consequences for the patient and his environment.'

The history of psychosomatic medicine alternated, pendulum-fashion from an organicist to a psychologically minded position. Such conditions as hypochondriasis (disorder under the costal arch) or hysteria (the wandering womb) presumed an underlying organic abnormality accounting for mental changes; this exemplified by *Thomas Sydenham* in the 17th century. A few years earlier *King James* I had written ascribing demon possession as the cause of psychological symptoms, and he was following a tradition firmly established in the Middle Ages. *Descartes* [1649], describing the engineer (the soul) inside the engine (the body) represented the philosophical dichotomy between body and mind in its clearest form [*Zilborg and Henry*, 1941], and this 'Cartesian dichotomy' has resulted in the separation of concepts of body and mind. Many authors have propounded a unitary concept of man, a holistic approach. Others such as *Popper and Eccles* [1977] in their book *The Self and Its Brain* are more prepared to take a tricotomous position with three interacting forms of ultimate reality: mind, body and self.

The concept *psychosomatic* was introduced by *Heinroth* [1818], but it was not until the 1930s that it became popular and a theoretical school within medicine developed with a largely psycho-analytic orientation. From this basis, *Dunbar* [1946] considered that certain specific personality profiles occurred with psychosomatic illnesses which included fracture, hypertension, coronary occlusion, angina, rheumatic heart disease, cardiac arrythmias, rheumatoid arthritis and diabetes. *Alexander* [1952] argued that it was not personality characteristics that account for the disease, but the presence of unresolved conflict. Powerful, but negative emotion, when frustrated from gaining expression, was converted into physiological disturbance, often autonomic in nature, with resultant physical illness. *Alexander's* list of psychosomatic diseases included bronchial asthma, ulcerative colitis, neuro-dermatitis, thyrotoxicosis and peptic ulcer, as well as rheumatoid arthritis and essential hypertension, to which *Dunbar* had already drawn attention.

Extant are many theories linking mind and body in the genesis of illness, of which some currently important are listed in table II. The *Cluster Theory* was described by *Hinkle and Wolff* [1957] who demonstrated that episodes of illness were not scattered at random through a population, but that they clustered with certain people having a greater risk of being ill than others; those who had major illnesses were more likely also to have minor illnesses; those who had illnesses in one system had an increased risk of illnesses in other systems; those who had somatic disease had more emotional and psychological symptoms, and clustering also occurred in time so that it was usual for the illnesses an individual suffered from to be concentrated within a period of perhaps 5–10 years.

Engel [1967] and others described the *giving-up, given-up complex*. Those with this attitude of hopelessness in the face of adversity were considered to be more likely to develop certain serious somatic illnesses. The features of the complex are as follows: (1) an affect of helplessness and hopelessness; (2) loss of self-esteem; (3) loss of gratification in relationships and roles; (4) disruption of the normal sense of continuity between the past, present and future, and (5) painful remembering of times when self-esteem was lowered.

The pathoplastic effect of *adverse life events* was studied by *Rahe* et al. [1967], who constructed a scale for life-changes (significant life events). Illness or clusters of illnesses tended to follow immediately after a cluster-year of life-changes; more severe illnesses were preceded by cluster-years of higher life-change magnitude. *Paykel* [1979] has developed research into the associations between adverse life events and various psychological and physical illnesses. The *experience of loss* has been investigated as a significant predictor of illness. For example, *Parkes* et al. [1969] found a sig-

Table II. Some current psychosomatic theories

---
1 Cluster theory [*Hinkle and Wolff,* 1957]
2 Affect of hopelessness – giving-up given-up complex [*Schmale and Iker,* 1966; *Engel,* 1967]
3 Adverse life events [*Rahe* et al., 1967]
4 Experience of loss [*Parkes* et al., 1969]
5 Alexithymia [*Nemiah and Sifneos,* 1970]
6 Type A behaviour pattern [*Friedman and Rosenman,* 1971]
7 Stress of life [*Selye,* 1956]
8 Last straw phenomenon [*Bennet,* 1970]
---

nificantly increased risk of death amongst widows in the 6 months immediately following their bereavement; they were also at greater risk for the development of serious illnesses and sought medical help more frequently.

The term *alexithymia* has been introduced by *Sifneos* to describe certain patients suffering from psychosomatic illnesses. These people show a marked difficulty in expressing their emotions in appropriate words; they only describe physical symptoms and do not introspect on the associated feelings. These patients do not describe fantasy and cannot recall their dreams; it is considered that their inability to express emotions leads to misdirection of libidinal activity with consequent physical damage [*Nemiah and Sifneos,* 1970]. *Friedman and Rosenman* [1971] related the behavioural characteristics of a large sample of normal men in California with the subsequent development of coronary artery disease. They considered that those healthy subjects demonstrating a *type A behaviour pattern,* characterised by competitive striving, aggressiveness, hostility and continuous working to time limits, were more likely to develop ischaemic heart disease. Evidence has been collected, especially by *Selye* [1956], to show an association between stress and the causation of disease. *Selye* considers that *stress* is the non-specific physiological response of the body to any demand made upon it – a stress reaction. *Bennet* [1970] ascribed the *last straw phenomenon* to those people living in Bristol whose houses were flooded, who experienced a higher cancer rate in the subsequent year. It was thought that these people were already prone to develop cancer but the acute stress accelerated their illness and death.

Is Neurosis Associated with Premature Mortality?

The term neurosis was introduced by *Cullen* in 1784 and has had extremely variable usage since that time [*Cullen,* 1784; *Sims,* 1985a]. It can be used, in an epidemiological sense, to include that large number of conditions which conform with the definition in the 9th Revision of the International Classification of Diseases: 'Neurotic disorders are mental disorders without any demonstrable organic basis in which the patient may have considerable insight and has unimpaired reality testing, in that he usually does not confuse his morbid subjective experiences and fantasies with external reality' [World Health Organization, 1977; *Sims,* 1984]. Such symptoms comprise over 90% of the psychiatric diagnoses amongst new attenders for a new complaint in general practice (Office of Population Censuses and Surveys, 1974); about 60% of those attending psychiatric out-patient clinics for the first time [*Sims and Salmons,* 1975]; and about 21% of those admitted as in-patients to psychiatric wards of a district general hospital [*Zigmond and Sims,* 1983]. When one considers that perhaps a sixth of all new attendances in general practice are for primarily psychological disturbance, then the frequency of neuroses and the resultant disturbances they cause are of considerable importance [*Shepherd and Clare,* 1981]. In this chapter the term neurosis is used in this epidemiological sense rather than having any psychodynamic, behavioural or phenomenological implications.

In epidemiological study, mortality is the 'hardest' information that is available when one considers the very 'soft' diagnosis of neurosis [*Sims,* 1984]. Since the beginning of psychiatric statistics in 1841 [*Farr,* 1841], it has been recognized that there is a considerably increased mortality rate for psychiatric in-patients. Initially, this increased mortality was especially from tuberculosis and gastro-intestinal infections, and of mental illnesses organic brain disease has been found to have the worst prognosis [*Eastwood* et al., 1982]. A markedly increased rate has however been described for many different psychiatric disorders in many types of treatment environment [*Sims,* 1982].

When the mortality specifically associated with neurosis is examined, there is of course no disturbance to the vital function and neurosis is not lethal of itself. Neurosis is very rarely invoked as a *cause of death* in death certification; for example, there were no deaths in 1981 recorded for neurosis (ICD 300). When observed deaths are compared with those expected in the follow-up of a sample of patients previously diagnosed as suffering from neurosis a variable, but usually significantly increased, relative risk is found. *Babigian and Odoroff* [1969] looked at those who died amongst the Monroe County Case Register and found the relative risk of death for neuroses to be 2.0 times the risk for the general population for males, and 1.8 times that for females. *Innes and Millar* [1970], in a case register in Scotland, found the mortality risk for neurosis to be 1.1 times that of the general population, and therefore not significantly increased. *Keehn* et al. [1974] followed up US army veterans discharged medically for psychoneurosis in 1944 and found a relative risk of 1.4 for males only. We found a relative risk of 1.7 when a sample of previously treated neurotic in-patients were followed up about 11 years later [*Sims and Prior,* 1978].

When conditions within neurosis are examined, a significant excess mortality due to death by unnatural causes was found in a 35-year follow-up after admission for panic disorder [*Coryell* et al., 1982]. Suicide accounted for 20% of the deaths and was more common than in a comparison group suffering from primary depression. A similar 42-year follow-up of women suffering from Briquet's syndrome revealed no evidence of excess mortality [*Coryell*, 1981a]. When those patients with more severe neurotic disorders are followed up, they are found to experience an increased premature mortality. Suicide and accidental death are considerably increased amongst these patients, and there is an excess of deaths from natural causes. Amongst these deaths from natural causes there is some evidence to incriminate arteriosclerotic disorders [*Sims and Prior*, 1980]. Neurotic in-patients are exposed to an increased toxicity from cigarette smoke and this may be a factor in the arteriosclerotic deaths from natural causes amongst the previously treated neurotic group [*Salmons and Sims*, 1981]. The increased mortality for neurosis is not explained by confusion over the term *depression*. Those neurotic patients who subsequently die are more likely to have suffered from a more severe degree of neurosis at the time of initial treatment [*Sims and Rudge*, 1979].

Suicide and accidental death are the most consistent causes of the excess mortality in psychiatric patients in general, and amongst neurotic disorders specifically. In an extensive review of psychiatric conditions predisposing to suicide, *Miles* [1977] came to the conclusion that neurosis showed a markedly increased rate, with perhaps 5% of patients diagnosed as suffering from neurosis or personality disorder subsequently dying by suicide. Whilst obsessive compulsive neurosis is found to have a lower suicide risk at follow-up, neurotic depression or psychopathic personality has a considerably increased risk [*Coryell*, 1981b]. In our study of 1,482 patients treated for neurosis in three hospitals and followed-up at a mean of 10.9 years after discharge, 139 patients (9.4% of the whole sample) had died. 60 of the deaths were reported to the coroner; 10% of all deaths were due to suicide and a further 10% recorded as accidental death [*Sims and Prior*, 1978].

Various psychosomatic and psychological hypotheses have been used to explain the increased mortality from neuroses [*Sims*, 1978]. It seems unlikely that the mortality is accounted for simply by missed organic diagnoses. Physical conditions resulting in death, and neurosis may be linked in the following ways: (1) Neurotic patients may be liable to an increased exposure to known physical causes of disease or death, e.g. tobacco, alcohol, dangerous driving. (2) For a given level of environmental exposure, neurotic patients may have an increased susceptibility to develop physical illness (psychosomatic disease). (3) With any given physical disease, neuroticism may have an adverse effect upon outcome.

Some of the psychosomatic explanations are included in table II. Psychosomatic theory for mortality requires a sequence from a morbid emotional state, behaviour pattern or personality structure to the development of a debilitating physical condition in which death may occur suddenly or gradually but undoubtedly prematurely. An important consideration is whether strong emotion, whether of fear, rage, grief or joy, can ever precipitate sudden death [*Elkinton*, 1971]. It has been proposed that extreme parasympathetic stimulation [*Burrell*, 1963] or extreme or prolonged sympathetico-adrenal discharge may lead to spontaneous ventricular fibrillation or long-standing vaso-constriction and reduction of blood volume [*Cannon*, 1942]. In addition to the listed theories in table II, it is suggested that an increased *severity* of neurosis is associated with greater predilection for death both from natural and unnatural causes [*Sims and Rudge*, 1979], and also that neurotic patients have a markedly increased likelihood of suffering accidents and of experiencing accidental death.

What is Accident Proneness?

The topic of accident proneness and its relevance for medicine has been excellently reviewed by *Connolly* [1981], who considers that 'the least assailable conclusions' are: '(1) There are accident repeaters but inequality of exposure is difficult to exclude as causal; (2) the repeating is possibly prolonged in a very small number of people; however, repeaters are mostly an ever-changing group and their identification would not lower accident rates by much; (3) the influence of age, training, experience, environment, drink, drugs, and physical disability is greater than those of factors such as fatigue and shift change; (4) psychological testing has not yet been very helpful.'

The term accident proneness was introduced by *Farmer and Chambers* [1939] who alleged that 'previous statistical investigations have shown that industrial workers exposed to risk were unequal in their liability to sustain accidents and that this unequal liability was a relatively stable phenomenon manifesting itself in different periods of exposure and in different kinds of accident'. They considered that this proneness was intrapersonal rather than environmental. Accident has been defined by *Arbous and Kerrich* [1951]: 'In a chain of events, each of which is planned or controlled, there occurs an unplanned event which, being the result of some non-adjusted act on the part of an individual, variously caused, may or may not result in injury.' They therefore make a clear distinction between the person who has the accident and the person who has the injury, who in some instances of course will be the same person. *Freud* [1925] considered that some accidents were unconsciously motivated, and *Menninger* [1938] developed this theory to explain 'purposive accident' in which unconscious self-destructive wishes found fulfillment. In the first systematic study of minor accidents, *Greenwood* et al. [1919] considered that amongst female munition workers there was unequal liability to accidents.

There has been considerable research subsequently into the characteristics of those experiencing higher rates of accident in terms of early development, personality characteristics, intellectual assessment, and experience of significant life events. Road traffic accidents have been studied in particular detail, and especially the drivers of public transport vehicles. However, in many ways these latter are an unsatisfactory sample for study as they tend to be preselected for low accident rate. Comparing taxi drivers in a high accident group with those rarely experiencing accidents, *Tillman and Hobbs* [1949] found that the former significantly more often had divorced parents, truancy and disciplinary problems at school, a history of being fired, frequent absences without leave during military service, and significantly more often admitted sexual promiscuity and bootlegging on the job. *Dalton* [1964] has claimed that women are more likely to experience accidents in the 8 days of the pre-menstrual and menstrual period than at other times of their cycle. The characteristics of accident-repeating children have been studied, and according to *Jones* [1980] there is a need to investigate the characteristics of the family as well as the personality and environment of the child.

There have been many reports critical of the methodology employed to substantiate *accident proneness,* and casting doubt on its existence as a significant phenomenon [*Haddon* et al., 1964]. From such studies it appears that the longer the interval between the periods studied the smaller the correlation for accidents happening to the same individuals. 'Examination of accident-repeaters over a lengthy period indicates that they are members of a club which is constantly changing its membership. New people are added, while long-standing members cease to qualify' [*Reason*, 1974]. More recently, the association between accidents and recent *experience, life-change,* and *life-events* has been explored [*Holmes and Rahe,*

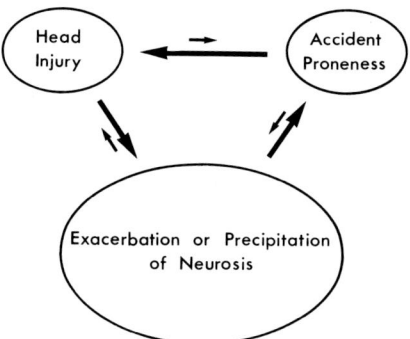

Fig. 1. Links between accident proneness, head injury and neurosis.

1967]. In many studies carried out in different cultures there has been found a significant association between accident or serious illness and increased life changes in the 6 months preceding. *Connolly* [1981] reported that men who experienced an accident whilst they were entirely alone described an excess of life-events in the 6 months preceding the accident. He concludes that there is at least a temporary increase in risk of accidental injury when life happenings cluster. Others have considered that accident proneness is not necessarily a permanent state of the individual but may well represent a temporary phase [*Selzer* et al., 1968].

Links between Accident Proneness and Neurosis

The three terms which form the title of this chapter may be seen as a triangle of inter-relationships; each having a possible effect on either of the other two. These relationships are shown in figure 1. The usual question is whether a neurotic reaction or a more consistent state of neuroticism is a factor in promoting accident proneness; however, it should also be queried as to whether the individual's experience of repeated accidents provokes neurotic reaction and resultant inappropriate behaviour.

According to *Guilford* [1973] there is a correlation between accidents in the home and automobile accidents, and these correlate with various demographic, attitudinal, physiological and cognitive characteristics of the subjects. These include a link between accidents and emotional instability, hypochondriasis, nervousness, the feeling of a need for freedom and lack of self-reliance. These findings would appear to support the concept of accident proneness associated with neuroticism. In a study of fatal accidents among car drivers, *MacDonald* [1964] found that those drivers with a psychiatric record were over-represented by more than 30 times the expected rate for the general population. *Schaffer and Fisher* [1974] found the personality profiles of fatally injured drivers to have been highly abnormal, and *Selzer* et al. [1968] found that drivers of vehicles who died as a result of their accidents showed significantly more symptoms of mental illness before their accident than a control group.

Drivers in single-car accidents were considered retrospectively to have shown significantly more psychopathology than those drivers in multiple-car accidents [*Schmitt* et al., 1972]. Psychiatric disturbance included anxiety, depression, alcohol abuse and impulsive acting-out behaviour. In a study of accident and injury reports from a large state mental hospital, *Abbott* [1978] considered that social disorganisation was the intervening variable in the hypothesis that crowding leads to violent injury.

In a recent study comparing 100 psychiatric patients with 100 carefully matched physically ill patients, despite a very much larger consumption of psychotropic drugs and a higher proportion of alcohol abusers in the psychiatric group, no significant differences were found between the two groups of patients with respect to accident and traffic code infringements [*Armstrong and Whitlock,* 1980]. Amongst the psychiatric patients no specific diagnostic group was associated with a higher accident liability apart from alcoholism.

In a study carried out in New Zealand, 150 suicide attempters, 100 drivers involved in automobile crashes and 200 controls randomly selected from the general population were compared on a number of variables and multivariate analyses applied to the data. Factors broadly associated with neurosis such as depression, neuroticism, social alienation and excessive amounts of undesirable life events with undesirable outcomes were significantly associated with suicidal behaviour but not with either the accident or control subjects. This large study, therefore, does not support a marked association between neurosis and accident proneness [*Isherwood* et al., 1982]. In an American study an attempt was made to develop a questionnaire to identify drivers who were highly susceptible to traffic accidents; this study demonstrated a relationship between life events, subjective stress and road accidents [*Selzer and Vinokur,* 1975].

In aviators, obsessive-compulsive personality has been identified as a precursor to accident proneness [*Banta and Kosnosky,* 1978]. In a single case study these authors identified perfectionistic and obsessional traits in a pilot of otherwise normal health and personality and they considered that there was evidence to ascribe his flying accident to these personality characteristics.

That the experience of repeated accidents should result in neurotic or inappropriate behaviour is in accord with theories of learned helplessness, as propounded by *Seligman* [1975] 'Learned helplessness can provide a model for understanding *reactive* depression, depression caused by environmental rather than internal events' [*Miller* et al., 1977]. Learned helplessness is the term introduced to describe what happens when prior exposure to uncontrollable aversive experiences interferes with escape and avoidance learning. This phenomenon has been demonstrated in a large number of animal experiments: whereas an animal without prior experience will try to escape from a noxious stimulus; when a similar animal has been exposed to this stimulus and prevented from escaping, on being subsequently allowed to escape during stimulus, it fails to do so. It is this mode of passive acceptance of circumstances – the tyranny of inevitability – which is comparable between the experimental description of learned helplessness and neurotic depression. The other aspect is that the noxious stimuli are seen as being outside the individual's control. In this sense the neurotic sees outside events as being accidents rather than in any way wholly or partially amenable to control, avoidance or prevention.

Links between Accident Proneness and Head Injury

The obvious association to investigate is that, if there are such people as *accident prone* individuals, amongst the physical damage to which they are more liable will be included *head injuries;* that is, unless there are specific protective factors for the head, those who have more accidents will also have more head injuries. This was the contention of the lobby for the introduction of crash helmets for motor cyclists, as demonstrated in the research of *Jamieson and Kelly* [1973] finding that adult civilian head injury victims were characterised by their youth, a previous history of anti-social behaviour, a higher rate of domestic and industrial accidents, and a higher incidence of disturbances in family life than non-injured individuals from a similar social group. The reverse association may also pertain; that is, that head injury increased the liability of an individual to other accidents through mechanisms such as impaired coordination and clumsiness; through loss of confidence in activities requiring skill and coordination.

Much of the evidence linking increased liability to accidents with head injury has been based on studies of accidents in children. Although individual behavioural characteristics are very important, family problems, difficulties in the relationships between the parents, and the health of parents are highly relevant [*Plionis*, 1976]. It is of course also very important to discriminate those cases where injury was truly accidental from non-accidental injury due to child abuse.

A random sample of 109 delinquent children referred to a juvenile court were compared with 109 non-delinquent children with similar demographic characteristics from Newhaven, Conn., USA. An evaluation of the medical history of each child in the study was made using the child's hospital record. Perinatal factors did not differentiate the two groups but the delinquent group had clustering of hospital contacts before age 4, and between the ages of 14 and 16; there was considered to be an interaction of developmental factors and parental inadequacies accounting for this. It was considered that early accidents and injuries, perhaps resulting from parental inadequacy, may have contributed to central nervous system dysfunction, which further aggravated the child's difficulties with impulse control and social adaptation [*Lewis and Shanock*, 1977]. In an Irish study, delinquent boys aged 10–16 gave a history of significant head injury with loss of consciousness and admission to hospital for more than 48 h in 7% of the sample compared with 4% of a control group who were not delinquent [*Barnes and O'Gorman*, 1978]. *Brown and Davidson* [1978] demonstrated an association between increased accident risk to children of 458 women living in an inner London area, and the presence of psychiatric disturbance (usually depression) and working-class status for the mothers. Whilst these authors in London had concentrated upon the mental state of the mother, *Jones* [1980] has commented upon the characteristics of the child who experiences repeated accidents; it was considered that the child with a suceptible personality had a tendency for accident repetition due to a breakdown in adjustment to a stressful environment.

Head injury increases the likelihood of certain deliberate and accidental forms of harmful behaviour; for example, suicide is very considerably increased among head-injured patients accounting for up to 14% of all deaths, and becoming increasingly frequent with the length of time elapsed since injury [*Achte and Anttinen*, 1963]. Behaviour disturbance commonly follows head injury in children, this consisting of restless overactivity intractableness and explosive outbursts of emotion. These characteristics predispose to further injury. The psychosocial sequelae of head injury due to boxing have included a chronic amnesic state, progressive dementia, morbid jealousy and rage reactions with uncontrolled outbursts of anger and violence [*Johnson*, 1969]; such individuals are further liable to accidental injury due to their impaired coordination and these outbursts of violence. Head injury results in a reduced tolerance for alcohol, and, as there is an association between alcohol abuse and situations which predispose to head injury (acute intoxication, chronic alcohol dependence syndrome, sequelae of boxing, etc.), this reduced tolerance, with continued overindulgence and frequenting the social milieu in which violence occurs may lead to further accidental injury.

The Link between Head Injury and Neurosis

This is perhaps the most contentious of the linkages in the hypothesized triangle of figure 1. Does head injury provoke an exacerbation or precipitation of neurotic disorder? Can neurosis as well as leading to an increased premature mortality also result in increased liability to head injury?

Characteristic of the numerical association between head injury and neurosis is a study reported by *Smith* [1979] conducted using the data of the West Virginia Workmen's Compensation Fund. 60 cases referred for psychiatric evaluation comprising 15 cases from each of four age groups between the ages of 18 and over 56 were investigated for both site of injury and psychiatric diagnosis. *Head injury,* with 18% of the sample, represented the second largest group, following *injury to the back* (43%). The majority of these subjects with injury-related psychiatric impairment suffered from *neurotic disorder* (58%), usually anxiety or depression. However, this 'guilt by association' by no means proves a causal linkage.

Mental disorders secondary to head injury are influenced by physiological, psychological and environmental factors [*Bond*, 1983]. If a distinction is made between mild injuries and those that are of moderate or severe degree, then the *post-concussion syndrome* and *accident neurosis* are characteristic of the former whilst *reactive depression,* often associated with the impairment of performance and loss of status thus engendered, frequently follows the latter. Psychological symptoms are extremely common following mild closed head injuries, even without loss of consciousness [*Miller*, 1961]. Men are twice as often affected as women; symptoms are much commoner with a work injury than in any other situation, and are more common with a large or nationalised industry than a smaller firm or if the patient is self-employed. The so-called *post-concussion syndrome* comprises the symptoms of headache, dizziness and emotional lability following head injury with concussion [*Ota*, 1969]; depression and lethargy are the commonest affective symptoms to occur. These symptoms either bear no relation to the degree of physical injury at all or may in fact even show an inverse relationship. This might suggest that the symptoms are more associated with psychological reaction than minimal degrees of brain damage. If physical symptoms are complained of in the absence of physical signs for more than a year after injury, then *accident neurosis* is considered to be present.

Trimble [1981] in his comprehensive study of *post-traumatic neurosis*, considered that 'neurotic symptoms are not only the prerogative of the mildly injured'. Neither the course nor aetiology has been proved to be associated with compensation. 'Psychogenesis' should not be too readily accepted as a cause for post-traumatic neurosis. Aetiology is clearly highly complex, and simplistic explanations of symptoms and behaviour are likely to be incorrect. In particular, obsessive-compulsive neurosis has been reported following head injury [*McKeon* et al., 1984] and it is likely that head injury exerts its pathogenetic effect through physical mechanisms producing heightened emotional arousal rather than as a perceived stress.

There seems to be an association between involvement in major catastrophe and the subsequent experience of neurotic reaction [*Sims*, 1985b]. Thus, when a group of victims who were geographically, and hence psychologically, involved in a major disaster but not seriously physically injured themselves were compared with a matched sample of accident and emergency attenders not involved in a major disaster, it was found that those involved had a great deal more time off work subsequently than the control group, who had in fact had more time off work due to sickness prior to their accident [*Sims* et al., 1979].

There certainly seems to be an association between head injury and the subsequent appearance of apparently neurotic symptoms. However, the aetiological questions remain. Are these symptoms organically determined? [*Taylor and Bell*, 1966]. Is it a post-traumatic reaction exacerbated because of the importance of the functions of the brain and the fears thereby promoted by their threatened loss in the patient? Is it associated with the expectation of compensation, or illness behaviour? Does the experience of involvement in disaster contribute? Perhaps many of these mechanisms are relevant, but *Lishman* [1973] has concluded: 'The evidence remains overwhelming that the *long-continued* "post-traumatic syndrome" rests principally on psychogenic mechanisms.' Clearly, the circumstances of the accident are important as also is the premorbid personality of the individual. *Lishman* [1978] has listed the aetiological factors in psychiatric disturbance after head injury as follows: (1) mental constitution; (2) premorbid personality; (3) emotional impact of injury; (4) emotional repercussions of injury; (5) environmental factors; (6) compensation and litigation; (7) response to intellectual impairments; (8) the development of epilepsy; (9) amount of brain damage incurred, and (10) location of brain damage incurred. These factors are of course operative to a varying degree in different individuals and it is often quite impossible to differentiate physiogenic from psychogenic causes.

In some series, neurotic disabilities have been the commonest psychiatric sequelae after head injury [*Ota,* 1969]. Somatic complaints are extremely common including headache and dizziness; psychological symptomes include hypochondriasis, depression, tension and anxiety, often phobic and obsessional symptoms, conversion hysteria, neurasthenia with inertia, irritability and hyperacusis. 'Change of personality' has frequently been described after severe head injury and may be both a neurotic sequel of head injury and also, through resultant change with deterioration in consistent behaviour, a cause of subsequent accidents and head injury. Other symptoms secondary to head injury may also predispose to neurotic reaction, for example, the loss of libido that is frequently associated with head injury such as in the *punch drunk syndrome.*

There is a clear association between the diagnosis of severe degrees of neurotic disorder and the subsequent development of alcohol and drug dependence [*Sims,* 1975]. Those who abuse alcohol or psychotropic drugs increase the likelihood of head injury either during acute intoxication or more chronic states of inebriation. From general practice records, for example, problem drinkers had a substantially higher number of medical symptoms; they consulted their doctor and attended casualty departments more frequently than a control group; they had more accidents and more marital and social problems [*Buchan* et al., 1981]. In a study from Sweden where alcohol-related deaths were investigated in a series of 199 male deaths, accidental death was only found amongst the alcohol-related group [*Petersson* et al., 1982]. Similarly, drug addicts may be involved in crimes of violence and are more likely to be the victims of homicide; the mortality risk is about 9% after 6 years of known addiction [*Thorley* et al., 1977].

There would thus appear to be two important mechanisms whereby those with neurotic disorder may be more liable to head injury. The first is the abuse of psychopharmacological agents, as described above, resulting in impaired coordination and increased risk taking. The second is the disturbance in social relationships which occurs with neurotic disorders. In a small minority of sufferers, this may result in physical violence with consequent injury to the subject. Disturbance of marriage, and of family and work relationships are extremely common amongst those experiencing neurotic disorder.

Conclusions

A triangle of inter-relationships has been hypothesized. Do these relationships actually exist?; in which direction do the arrows go?; how common are these linkages – are they epidemiologically important? The evidence quoted above is mostly of a tentative rather than conclusive nature, and considerable research is required to clarify the situation. Accident proneness remains a disputed concept although it appears that certain individuals do become more liable to accidents for a period of time. It is difficult to know how long is the duration of this increased risk, perhaps it is a cluster of approximately a few years. Neurosis also is a much-disputed concept but has some usefulness in making a distinction from other psychiatric disorders. Amongst head injuries there does definitely seem to be an association with neurosis. This is clearly a very common sequel to head injury; there are therefore social, prophylactic and therapeutic implications for the management of head injury. There is a need for future research both to elucidate the linkages and also to investigate the therapeutic possibilities.

References

Abbott, A.: Accident and its correlates in a psychiatric hospital. Acta psychiat. scand. *57:* 36–48 (1978).
Achte, K.A.; Anttinen, E.E.: Suizide bei Hirngeschädigten des Krieges in Finnland. Fortschr. Neurol. Psychiat. *31:* 645–667 (1963).
Alexander, F.: Psychosomatic medicine. Its principles and applications (Allen & Unwin, London 1952).
Arbous, A.G.; Kerrich, J.E.: Biometrics *7:* 340 (1951).

Armstrong, J.L.; Whitlock, F.A.: Mental illness and road traffic accidents. Aust. N. Z. J. Psychiat. *14:* 53–60 (1980).
Babigian, H.M.; Odoroff, C.L.: The mortality experience of a population with psychiatric illness. Am. J. Psychiat. *126:* 470–480 (1969).
Banta, G.R.; Kosnosky, D.P.: Case report of an obsessive-compulsive personality. A precursor to accident proneness. Aviation, Space envir. Med. *49:* 827–828 (1978).
Barnes, J.; O'Gorman, N.: Some medical and social features of delinquent boys. J. Irish med. Ass. *71:* 19–20 (1978).
Bennet, G.: Bristol floods 1968. Controlled survey of effects on health of local community disaster. Br. med. J. *iii:* 454–458 (1970).
Bond, M.R.: Head injury and changes in brain function secondary to electroconvulsive therapy and psychosurgery; in Lader, Handbook of psychiatry: mental disorders and somatic illness (Cambridge University Press, Cambridge 1983).
Brown, G.W.; Davidson, S.: Social class, psychiatric disorder of mother and accidents to children. Lancet *i:* 378–381 (1978).
Buchan, I.C.; Buckley, E.G.; Deacon, G.L.; Irvine, R.; Ryan, M.P.: Problem drinkers and their problems. J. R. Coll. gen. Pract. *31:* 151–153 (1981).
Burrel, R.J.W.: The possible bearing of curse death and other factors in Bantu culture on the etiology of myocardial infarction; in James & Keyes, Henry Ford Hospital International Symposium. The etiology of myocardial infarction (Churchill, London 1963).
Cannon, W.B.: 'Voodoo' death. Psychosom. Med. *19:* 182–190 (1957).
Connolly, J.: Accident proneness. Br. J. Hosp. Med. *26:* 470–481 (1981).
Connolly, J.: J. psychosom. Res. (1981).
Coryell, W.: Diagnosis – specific mortality: primary unipolar depression and Briquet's syndrome (somatisation disorder). Archs gen. Psychiat. *38:* 939–942 (1981a).
Coryell, W.: Obsessive compulsive disorder and primary unipolar depression: comparisons of background, family history, course and mortality. J. nerv. ment. Dis. 169: 220–224 (1981b).
Cullen, W.: First lines in the practice of physic, vol.I–IV (Elliot, Cadell, Edinburgh 1784).
Curran, D.; Partridge, M.: Psychological medicine; 6th ed. (Churchill Livingstone, Edinburgh 1969).
Dalton, K.D.: The premenstrual syndrome (Heinemann, London 1964).
Descartes, R.: Les passions de l'âme; in Descartes, Philosophical writings (1649). Trans. K. Smith (MacMillan, London 1952).
Dunbar, F.: Emotions and bodily change. A survey of literature on psychosomatic interrelationships; 3rd ed. (Columbia University Press, New York 1946).
Eastwood, M.R.; Stiasny, S.; Meier, H.M.: Mental illness and mortality. Compreh. Psychiat. *23:* 377–385 (1982).
Elkinton, J.R.: Scared to death? Ann. intern. Med. *74:* 789–790 (1971).
Engel, G.L.: The psychological setting of somatic disease: the giving-up-given-up complex, Proc. R. Soc. Med. *60:* 553–555 (1967).
Enoch, M.D.; Irving, G.: The Ganser syndrome. Acta psychiat. Scand. *48:* 213–222 (1962).
Farmer, E.; Chambers, E.G.: A study of accident proneness among motor drivers, report No. 84 (Industrial Health Research Board, London 1939).
Farr, W.: Report upon the mortality of lunatics. J. statist. Soc. *4:* 17–33 (1841).
Freud, S.: Collected papers, vol. 3 (Hogarth Press, London 1925).

Friedman, M.; Rosenman, R.H.: Type A behaviour pattern: its association with coronary heart disease. Ann. clin. Res. *3:* 300 (1971).

Ganser, S.J.: A peculiar hysterical state. Arch. Psychiat. NervKrankh. *30:* 633. Trans. Schorer 1965. Br. J. Criminol. 5: 120–126 (1898).

Granville-Grossman, K.: Mind and body; in Lader, Mental disorders and somatic illness. Handbook of psychiatry. vol. 2 (Cambridge University Press, Cambridge 1983).

Greenwood, M.; Woods, H.M.; Yule, G.U.: A report on the incidence of industrial accidents upon individuals with special reference to multiple accidents, report No. 4 (Industrial Fatigue Research Board, London 1919).

Guilford, J.S.: Prediction of accidents in a standardised home environment. J. appl. Psychol. *57:* 306–313 (1973).

Haddon, W.; Suchman, E.A.; Klein, D.: Accident research (Harper & Row, New York 1964).

Heinroth, J.C.: Lehrbuch der Störungen des Seelenlebens (Leipzig, 1818).

Hinkle, L.E.; Wolff, H.G.: The nature of man's adaptation to his total environment and the relation of this to illness. Archs intern. Med. *99:* 442–460 (1957).

Holmes, T.H.; Rahe, R.H.: The social readjustment rating scale. J. Psychosom. Res. *11:* 213–218 (1967).

Innes, G.; Millar, W.M.: Mortality among psychiatric patients. Scott. med. J. *15:* 143–148 (1970).

Isherwood, J.; Adam, K.S.; Hornblow, A.R.: Life event stress, psychosocial factors, suicide attempt and auto-accident proclivity. J. psychosom. Res. *26:* 371–383 (1982).

Jamieson, K.G.; Kelly, D.: Crash helmets reduce head injuries. Med. J. Aust. *ii:* 806–809 (1973).

Johnson, J.: Organic psychosyndromes due to boxing. Br. J. Psychiat. *115:* 45–53 (1969).

Jones, J.G.: The child accident repeater. A review. Clin. Pediatr. *19:* 284–288 (1980).

Keehn, R.J.; Goldberg, I.D.; Beebe, G.W.: Twenty four year mortality follow-up of army veterans with disability separations for psychoneurosis in 1944. Psychosom. Med. *36:* 27–46 (1974).

King James I.: Daemonologie, in form of a dialogue (Waldegrave, Edinburgh 1597); in Hunter, MacAlpine, Three hundred years of psychiatry, 1535–1860 (Oxford University Press, London 1963).

Latcham, R.W.; White, A.C.; Sims, A.C.: Ganser syndrome: the aetiological argument. J. Neurol. Neurosurg. Psychiat. *42:* 851–854 (1978).

Lewis, D.O.; Shanok, S.S.: Medical histories of delinquent and non-delinquent children: an epidemiological study. J. Psychiat. *134:* 1020–1025 (1977).

Lipowski, Z.J.: Psychosomatic medicine: an overview; in Hill, Modern trends in psychosomatic medicine, No. 3 (Butterworth, London 1976).

Lishman, W.A.: The psychiatric sequelae of head injury. A review. Psychol. Med. *3:* 304–318 (1973).

Lishman, W.A.: Organic psychiatry. The psychological consequences of cerebral disorder (Blackwell, Oxford 1978).

MacDonald, J.M.: Suicide and homicide by automobile. J. Am. Psychiat. *121:* 366–370 (1964).

McKeon, J.; McGuffin, P.; Robinson, P.: Obsessive-compulsive neurosis following head injury: A report of four cases. Br. J. Psychiat. *144:* 190–192 (1984).

Menninger, K.: Man against himself (Harcourt Brace & World Incorporated, New York 1938).
Miles, C.P.: Conditions predisposing to suicide. A review. J. nerv. ment. Dis. *164:* 231–246 (1977).
Miller, H.: Accident neurosis. Br. med. J. *1:* 919–925.
Miller, W.R.; Rosellini, R.A.; Seligman, M.E.: Depression: learned helplessness and depression; in Maser, Seligman, Psychopathology: experimental methods (Freeman, San Francisco 1977).
Nemiah, J.L.; Sifneos, P.E.: Affect and fantasy in patients with psychosomatic disorders; in Hill, Modern trends in psychosomatic medicine, No. 2 (Butterworth, London 1970).
Office of Population Censuses and Surveys: Morbidity statistics from general practice. Second National Study 1970–1971 (HMSO, London 1974).
Ota, Y.: Psychiatric studies on civilian head injuries; in Walker, Caveness, Critchley, The late effects of head injury (Thomas, Springfield 1969).
Parkes, C.M.; Benjamin, B.; Fitzgerald, R.G.: Broken heart. A statistical survey of increased mortality amount widowers. Br. med. J. *1:* 740–743 (1969).
Paykel, E.S.: Recent life events and clinical depression; in Gunderson, Rahe, Life stress and illness (Thomas, Springfield 1979).
Petersson, B.; Krantz, P.; Kristensson, H.: Trell, E.; Sternby, N.H.: Alcohol related death: a major contribution to mortality in urban middle aged men. Lancet *ii:* 1088–1090 (1982).
Plionis, E.M.: Family functioning and childhood accident occurrence. Am. J. Orthopsychiat. *47:* 250–263 (1976).
Popper, K.R.; Eccles, J.C.: The self and its brain (Springer, Berlin 1977).
Rahe, R.H.; McKean, J.D.; Arthur, R.J.: A longitudinal study of life-change and illness patterns. J. psychosom. Res. *10:* 355–366 (1967).
Reason, J.: New Society *27:* 445 (1974).
Salmons, P.H.; Sims, A.C.: Smoking profiles of patients admitted for neurosis. Br. J. Psychiat. *139:* 43–46 (1981).
Schmale, A.H.; Iker, H.P.: The affect of hopelessness and the development of cancer. I. Identification of uterine cervical cancer in women with atypical cytology. Psychol. Med. *28:* 714–721 (1966).
Schmidt, C.W.; Perlin, S.; Fisher, R.S.; Shaffer, J.W.: Characteristics of drivers involved in single car accidents – a comparative study. Archs gen. Psychiat. *27:* 800–803 (1972).
Seligman, M.E.: Helplessness (Freeman, San Francisco 1975).
Selye, H.: The stress of life (McGraw-Hill, New York 1956).
Selzer, M.L.; Rogers, J.E.; Kern, S.: Fatal accidents: the role of psychopathology, social stress and acute disturbance. Am. J. Psychiat. *124:* 1028–1036 (1968).
Selzer, M.L.; Vinokur, A.: Role of life events in accident causation. Ment. Hlth Soc. *2:* 36–54 (1975).
Shaffer, J.W.; Fisher, R.S.: Social adjustment profiles of fatally injured drivers. A replication and extension. Archs gen. Psychiat. *30:* 508–511 (1974).
Shepherd, D.M.; Clare, A.: Psychiatric illness in general practice; 2nd ed. (Oxford University Press, London 1981).
Sims, A.C.: Dependence on alcohol and drugs following treatment for neurosis. Br. J. Addiction *70:* 33–40 (1975).

Sims, A.C.: Hypotheses linking neuroses with premature mortality. Psychol. Med. 8: 255–263 (1978).
Sims, A.C.: Mortality in psychiatric patients; in Koranyi, Physical illness in the psychiatric patient (Thomas, Springfield 1982).
Sims, A.C.: Neurosis and mortality: investigating an association. J. psychosom. Res. 28: 353–362 (1984).
Sims, A.C.: Mental illness and urban disaster; in Freeman, Mental health and the environment (awaiting publication, 1985b).
Sims, A.C.: Neurosis 1784–1984. Two centuries of obfuscation (awaiting publication, 1985a).
Sims, A.C.: The pattern of mortality in severe neuroses. Br. J. Psychiat. 133: 299–305 (1978).
Sims, A.C.; Prior, M.P.: Arteriosclerosis-related deaths in severe neurosis. Compreh. Psychiat. 23: 181–185.
Sims, A.C.; Rudge, B.J.: Discriminators between neurotics who die and neurotics who live. Acta psychiat. scand. 59: 317–325 (1979).
Sims, A.C.; Salmons, P.H.: The severity of symptoms of psychiatric outpatients – use of the General Health Questionnaire in hospital and general practice patients. Psychol. Med. 5: 62–66 (1975).
Sims, A.C.; White, A.C.; Murphy, T.: Aftermath neurosis: Psychological sequelae of the Birmingham bombings in victims not seriously injured. Med. Sci. Law 19: 78–81 (1979).
Smith, R.S.: The psychiatrically-impaired injured worker. I. Background and data review. W. Va. med. J. 75: 154–158 (1979).
Sydenham, T.: Epistle to Dr. William Cole; in Robinson, Otridge, Hayes, Neuberg, The works of Thomas Sydenham with annotation by Wallis, 1788 (London 1681).
Taylor, A.R.; Bell, T.K.: Slowing of cerebral circulation after concussional head injury. A controlled trial. Lancet ii: 178–180 (1966).
Thorley, A.; Oppenheimer, E.; Stimson, G.V.: Clinic attendance and opiate prescription status of heroin addicts over a six year period. Br. J. Psychiat. 130: 565–569 (1977).
Tillmann, W.A.; Hobbs, L.E.: The accident prone automobile driver. Am. J. Psychiat. 106: 321 (1949).
Trimble, M.R.: Post-traumatic neurosis: from railway spine to the whiplash (Wiley, Chichester 1981).
Tsoi, W.F.: The Ganser syndrome in Singapore. A report of ten cases. Br. J. Psychiat. 123: 567–572 (1973).
Whitlock, F.A.: The Ganser syndrome. Br. J. Psychiat. 113: 19–29 (1967).
World Health organisation: International Statistical Classification of diseases, injuries and causes of death; 9th Revision (WHO, Geneva 1977).
Zigmond, A.S.; Sims, A.C.: The effect of the use of the International Classification of Diseases 9th Revision, upon hospital inpatient diagnoses. Br. J. Psychiat. 142: 409–413 (1983).
Zilboorg, G.; Henry, G.W.: A history of medical psychology (Morton, New York 1941).

Prof. A.C.P. Sims, MA, MD, FRC Psych., Department of Psychiatry,
St. James's University Hospital, Leeds LS9 7TF (UK)

4. Emotional Aspects of Cerebrovascular Disease

Peter Storey

St. George's and Springfield Hospitals, London, UK

Many risk factors have been identified in stroke illnesses. *Leonberg and Elliott* [1981] list the following: hypertension, diabetes mellitus, hyperlipidaemia, atherosclerotic disease, erythrocythaemia, stress, tobacco smoking, hyperuricaemia and obesity. Binge drinking of alcohol could be added to the list [Lancet, Editorial, 1983].

In the broadest (and best) sense of the word psychosomatic, we could consider emotional and personality factors as operative in several of their list of ten, and not just under the heading of 'stress'. For example, hypertension has links with personality and environmental stress, something which is discussed in more detail later. Tobacco smoking is certainly related to personality, and to emotional stress. Obesity has psychosocial aspects; and insofar as hyperlipidaemia and hyperuricaemia depend on what one eats, the same is true for them. Physical exercise is not mentioned by *Leonberg and Elliott*, although others consider it important, but it again depends largely on attitudes, interests and other psychosocial factors.

This article will not continue to labour these broader psychosomatic implications, as the point is obvious: that psychosocial factors not only largely determine how we live, but also how we fall ill and die. We will restrict ourselves to some of the emotional and cultural factors related to stroke illness (including subarachnoid haemorrhage) in predisposition, precipitation and emotional sequelae. As hypertension is the major risk factor known, it will first be considered separately.

Hypertension

Hypertension is such an important risk factor for strokes that it is worth briefly considering the evidence for the role of psychosocial factors in its genesis. The subject has very recently been reviewed by *Mann* [1984]. We will not consider animal experiments, nor transient rises of blood pressure in humans with emotional or other psychological stimuli, although there is vast literature on those subjects, but sketch in some of the main areas of research in which the psychogenesis of hypertension has been studied in man.

Anxiety and Hypertension

Interest was first focussed on findings that hypertensive patients were more anxious and 'neurotic' on questionnaire assessment than were other people [*Sainsbury,* 1964]. Later studies showed that this only applied to hypertensives attending hospital who knew the diagnosis, whereas subjects found by population screening, who were unaware of their blood pressure, were not more anxious or neurotic than the normotensives [*Kidson,* 1973; *Monk,* 1980]. Treatment with reserpine, which was common when the earlier studies were done, may also have led to anxiety or depressive symptoms [*Cochrane,* 1969]. One must remember too that doctors often take the blood pressure of people who complain of headache, a common anxiety and tension symptom, which is an added selection factor, as anxious people visit their doctor with more complaints generally than do others [British Medical Journal, 1976].

In his own study, which was part of a large trial of treatment in hypertension organised by the Medical Research Council, *Mann* [1984], found no relationship between psychiatric morbidity and diastolic blood pressure in 12,693 subjects, using the General Health Questionnaire (GHQ) [*Goldberg,* 1972]. There was an interesting fall during the course of the trial in the psychiatric morbidity which *was* recorded by the questionnaire: a fall which *Mann* attributed to the sessions with the nurse who regularly assessed each patient, and provided opportunities for discussion of problems and helpful support.

In summary, one can say that there is no good evidence linking hypertension to anxiety, or other neurotic symptoms as measured by questionnaire.

It should, however, be pointed out that despite these negative findings there is evidence that biofeedback aided relaxation techniques can lower blood pressure, in mild hypertension at least [*Patel* et al., 1981]. Further instruction in cognitive methods of stress management has recently been shown to be as effective as relaxation therapy [*Wadden,* 1984].

Depressive Illness and Hypertension

In an interesting paper, *Heine* [1970] described a small study in which it was found that patients in hospital with severe depressive illness had blood pressures higher than non-depressives, and that in patients with more than one depressive illness blood pressure rose with each episode, and was sustained at a higher level after clinical recovery. Blood pressure was thus correlated with the number of depressive attacks in some people. The rise only applied to systolic pressure, but the Framingham data [*Kannel*, 1983] show that systolic pressure predicts stroke as well as diastolic pressure.

Unexpressed Hostility and Hypertension

Another influential idea about the psychogenesis of hypertension, derived initially from psychoanalytic observations, has been that hypertension develops in people who are unable to express anger, but bottle it all up, appearing less assertive than normal. It is presumed that the undischarged rage leads to disturbances of, for example, adrenaline output and sympathetic nervous system activity, which leads in turn to hypertension.

Studies of larger populations using a questionnaire which attempts to assess the intensity of hostility, and whether it is directed inwardly or outwards to others (the Hostility and Direction of Hostility Questionnaire or HDHQ of *Foulds* [1965]) has not supported these claims of a relationship between feelings of anger and hypertension. *Mann* [1984], for example, found no such relation in 53 normotensives and 55 hypertensives.

The present author does not consider that the HDHQ can be said to measure exactly what needs to be measured, if the clinical concept of repressed anger is to be studied properly in relation to hypertension. It is, of course, extremely difficult to develop questionnaires for such complex concepts.

The evidence in favour of the association is not strong, and at present it seems to be best to regard it as unlikely, but not as disproven.

Type A Behaviour and Hypertension

'Type A' behaviour was described by *Friedman and Rosenman* [1959] as being a major risk factor in ischaemic heart disease. Rather curiously, its relationship with hypertension was not considered in their first paper, but has been in later studies by the same group and by other investigators. 'Type A' indicates the characteristics of intense sustained drive for achievement, and a continual involvement in competition and deadlines, both in work and other activities. Although strongly associated with ischaemic heart disease in many studies, the claimed relationship with hypertension is not marked. *Gianturco* et al. [1974] had interesting findings in this context, described later.

Cultural and Environmental Factors and Hypertension

This title covers many diverse approaches to the ways in which style of life, and in particular major disruptive changes, such as follow emigration, affect blood pressure. There is an extensive literature on the subject, reviewed by *Marmot* [1981].

It is well known that there are many societies around the world, mainly with simple rural patterns of life, but including hunter-gatherers, in which the average blood pressure is low by western standards, and in which there is no significant rise with age [*Henry and Cassel,* 1969]. It has also been shown that when such peoples emigrate to more developed countries or move to urban areas in their own country, blood pressure rises. Unfortunately, no one has been able to disentangle convincingly the possible effects of psychosocial stress from physical factors such as increased salt or saturated fat intake, although brave attempts have been made, and to the present writer the accumulating evidence is increasingly persuasive.

Studies of overcrowding in prisons, which represent a different type of ecological upheaval, have strongly suggested a relationship with hypertension. For example, *D'Atri* et al. [1981] showed that prisoners moved to a larger dormitory showed a rise in blood pressure compared to those left behind in a one-man cell. Whether or not the rise endures after leaving prison has not yet been established.

The working environment and 'occupational stress' are regarded by many people, doctors and laymen alike, as singularly relevant to hypertension, and at least one study provides rather strong evidence in support. *Cobb and Rose* [1973] found that air traffic controllers, who work under great pressure of time and responsibility, had higher blood pressures than other employees in the company, and that air traffic controllers show rises in blood pressure after starting the work which others, starting from a similar baseline but doing less demanding work, do not show. In addition, those who work at the busier air bases show greater rises. Although it was not possible to control for all possible factors, and differences in exercise or diet could still be relevant, this study is convincing.

Comment. Hypertension, which is the major known risk factor in stroke illnesses, has in the public mind been firmly associated with 'stress' for a long time. There is in fact less objective evidence to support the notion than many might suppose, perhaps because there are so many confounding factors for which it is difficult to allow. To the present author, the best evidence to date is that showing the effect of environmental and occupational factors as in the studies of overcrowding in prisons and of air traffic controllers. It is a striking clinical fact, however, that physicians who deal with hypertensive patients tell them to 'take it easy' in one way or another, whether or not those physicians are interested in basic psychosomatic ideas. They would possibly also be prepared to attribute a patient's deterioration to the fact that he had troubles at work at the same time that his wife had been in hospital, so that he had to visit her as well as look after the children in the evenings. This kind of stressful situation, so frequent in life, is difficult to pin down conceptually and translate into relevant and valid measuring scales.

Stroke Illnesses: Emotional Factors in Predisposition and Precipitation

Relatively little has been written on these subjects compared to hypertension and ischaemic heart disease, although it has always been known that strokes could be precipitated by emotional upheaval. For example, *Lidell* [1873] had a category of 'nervous apoplexy' to cover cases 'caused by terror or grief' in his monograph on various forms of stroke. Most of the articles published have produced evidence to support a psychosomatic link, as one might expect, but *Heyden* [1978], in a review of stress in arteriosclerotic disease, is very dismissive of such an approach and emphasises the difficulty of controlling for diet, exercise and other factors. He is also dismissive of speculations being accepted as fact.

As many of the articles reviewed consider both longer term predisposition and immediate precipitation, they are not rigorously separated here.

It is very difficult to distinguish, practically if not conceptually, between the psychogenesis of hypertension and any long-term psychogenic effects on predisposition to stroke which might exist, independent of hypertension. The easiest field to study is that of the immediate precipitation by emotional turmoil, but some evidence linking personality to stroke is mentioned later in this review.

Several studies have been influential, but to the writer unconvincing, in their attempts to link strokes to long-standing emotional factors. For example, *Ecker* [1954] said that before cerebral strokes there had been in many of his cases '... long-standing progressive difficulty in settling emotional problems'. It is, however, obvious that progressive but so far unrecognised atherosclerotic or hypertensive changes might be the cause of that 'progressive difficulty' well before the stroke which brings the patient to medical attention. The same possibility applies to several other papers with similar conclusions, and generally to the application of the concept of the 'giving up-given up' complex [*Schmale,* 1958].

A well-known paper of this type on both predisposition and precipitation in stroke illnesses was that by *Adler* et al. [1971]. This was a retrospective anamnestic study of 32 men who had 35 strokes. The authors believed that the patients demonstrated many personality features in common, especially a so-called 'pressured' pattern, very like that of the type A of *Friedman and Rosenman* [1959]. They also concluded that the strokes occurred in situations where the patient was reacting, mainly with anger and hopelessness, to his sense of failure to live up to his own standards, and to remain in control of things generally. Unfortunately, the study has serious drawbacks, and although suggestive, the findings cannot be accepted without reservation. No controls were interviewed, and the tape recordings used were not rated blind. In other words, there is no real evidence that these men differed importantly in personality from men who do not have strokes. In addition, as in the last paper mentioned, no allowance was made for the strong probability that many of these severely hypertensive men were failing to live up to their standards, and failing to maintain control, *because* of early ischaemic brain disease, rather than that the failure precipitated the strokes.

It is now widely accepted that there is an increased mortality and morbidity among surviving spouses after bereavement, or after other major life events. In fact, strokes do not seem to play much part in these increases, although ischaemic heart disease does. For example, the study by *Parkes* et al. [1969] showed absolutely no increase in cerebrovascular disease in the bereaved population compared to the expected rate. In studies of a different type of stress, *Nefzeger* [1970], following up people who had been prisoners of war, demonstrated the well-known increased mortality among those who had been prisoners of the Japanese. Strokes did not seem to play a part in this increase, although the population was perhaps too young at the time of follow-up to demonstrate any increase that might develop.

Many authors have commented on the increased mortality rate in people with psychiatric symptoms, but these studies do not show any particularly high incidence of stroke illness. In fact, *Sims* [1973] noted that patients with neurosis die from the same complaints as the general population. The much larger study of *Sims and Prior* [1978] had similar findings; namely that strokes appear among the causes of death, but not in large numbers. In some such studies strokes are, in fact, conspicuous by their absence, as, for example, in that by *Murphy and Brown* [1980].

Looking at more general 'life style' factors of the sort mentioned at the start of this article, a large study, following up more than 7,500 people, by *Salonen* et al. [1982] produced interesting results. They showed that strokes, myocardial infarction and early death were all more common in those who took less exercise (controlling for many other factors). However, this did not apply to levels of physical activity in leisure time but was related really to manual work. Now leisure time activity seems much more likely to be related to personality factors than is other physical activity, so these findings are, indirectly, against the importance of personality factors in this narrow field.

A small, but convincing, study was that by *Gianturco* et al. [1974]. They were seeking evidence for the frequency of type A personality [*Friedman and Rosenman,* 1959] in patients after stroke. They had 26 cases, free from confusion, dysphasia and so on, and 14 controls. They found type A personality mainly in those patients who had a previous history of ischaemic heart disease rather than in those with stroke alone. Those same patients were more likely to describe feelings of anger or anxiety in the period immediately before the stroke. They comment also that these stroke patients generally did not seem to have obvious problems in coping with anger, which is relevant to the concept of the importance of repressed hostility mentioned in the section on hypertension. The ordinary layman's view of 'apoplexy' of course, was that rage was likely to bring it on, an idea which has almost reached the level of folklore.

One study which found strongly positive associations between personality factors and stroke was that by *Carasso* et al. [1981]. They took 384 successive patients admitted to an emergency room with a diagnosis of cerebrovascular accident, and each was asked to anwer questions on a measure of type A personality. About 85% of the patients were found to have type A personality, an extremely high figure, with the incidence being somewhat higher in those with a past history of cardiovascular disease. They also found a high incidence of life events on the *Holmes and Rahe* [1967] scale; and in stroke patients without a previous history of cardiovascular disease there was a significant association between the life events score and the severity of the stroke. Confidence in this paper is weakened by the absence of any information about how many patients with confusion, dysphasia or other mental disabilities were included or excluded: a strange oversight.

Ecker [1954] and *Seidenberg and Ecker* [1954] discussed the role of emotional stress and individual psychopathology in strokes generally, drawing their examples mainly from subarachnoid haemorrhage. They believed that emotional stress could cause cerebral arterial spasm, which then led to the haemorrhage; but this approach is really invalidated by the fact that blood in the cerebrospinal space causes cerebral arterial spasm, rather than vice versa. Some of their cases did, however, show very convincing associations between immediate major emotional disturbance and strokes.

Similar evidence of immediate emotional precipitation of subarachnoid haemorrhage was published by *Storey* [1969, 1972], except that in those cases emotional precipitation was almost confined to those with normal angiograms. It was rare in aneurysm cases, and was confined to women. In a first series of 261 patients who were being seen as part of a follow-up study of subarachnoid haemorrhage, and in which no particular interest in mode of onset was at first taken, there were 30 patients with normal angiograms. They had been included as a kind of control group, as they are known to sustain little or no brain damage. In only 1 of the 231 aneurysm patients was an emotional precipitant described – she was watching a television news feature about a new plane on which she believed her son was flying when it exploded, and her haemorrhage followed in seconds. In 6 of 30 patients with normal angiograms, emotional precipitants were described, in 4 almost as dramatic as that just mentioned in the aneurysm case.

Equally interesting in the study was the finding that as a group those with subarachnoid haemorrhage and normal angiograms had a high incidence of psychiatric morbidity before as well as after the haemorrhage, and this condition – in which haemorrhage is thought to occur from microaneurysms on the meningeal vessels – seems to affect an emotionally vulnerable and neurotic group. These observations are, of course, quite different from those made about the more common stroke illnesses, and it should be noted that these patients are not hypertensive as are most stroke sufferers.

As a check on those unsystematic and largely retrospective findings, a small prospective study was done [*Penrose and Storey*, 1970], in which relatives were interviewed when patients were first admitted, before the results of angiography were known. The relatives described more emotional turmoil and more life events in those who turned out to have normal angiograms than in those with aneurysms.

In summary, there is no doubt – as there has never been – that strokes can be precipitated immediately by major emotional turmoil. There is, however, little evidence so far that personality or emotional factors can be linked with long-term predisposition to strokes (except for the small group of subarachnoid haemorhage patients with normal angiograms) independent of hypertension. As we have seen, the psychogenesis of hypertension and its relation to 'stress' is not so firmly established either. More life events studies are obviously desirable in this field, with careful attention to methodology.

Some Consequences of Strokes

Cerebrovascular accidents are not only a major cause of death, but also one of the most important causes of physical and mental disability. The suffering they cause is incalculable. In a chapter mainly devoted to the antecedents of stroke, it nevertheless seems appropriate to consider very briefly some of the consequences, concentrating on affective changes. Perceptual and intellectual loss will only be mentioned in passing.

No stroke can be lightly dismissed once it is recognised as such, even if it leaves no ill effects, because of the fear of recurrence. In fact, most strokes do lead to significant impairment; and, also, most single strokes are only episodes in a progressive illness.

Holbrook [1982] gives a good brief account of the stages through which most patients pass after a major stroke, and also considers the social consequences. The first stage she describes is that of shock and confusion, with anxiety and dread about disability and the loss of so much that makes life sweet. Next, the second stage in which high hopes of treatment develop, and fears are kept at bay by hope and denial. The third stage of 'realisation' brings anger and despair, and that increasing intensity of frustration which is central in the lives of stroke survivors. The third stage also brings depression, so characteristic of these patients. Many never reach the fourth stage of acceptance and adjustment, and one only has to be involved in the care of those with strokes to realise how difficult acceptance must be. In the series on which *Holbrook* bases her report, 41%

could not walk out of doors, and altogether two-thirds rarely or never went out. There were problems of loss of income, changes in daily life style, in the patterns of family relationships, in social life generally, and the loss of role which is such an important part of the problem.

Many other authors have written similarly, emphasising different aspects of the illness, from medical, nursing and social work viewpoints; and some patients have written of their experiences very eloquently [*Ritchie*, 1960]. Other authors have emphasised the specific disabilities in language, comprehension and perceptual problems, not forgetting the obvious and often gross motor and sensory loss. Loss of sexual abilities is also extremely common after strokes. Review of these and other subjects are given in the volume edited by *Benton* [1970]. Very good accounts of the difficulties caused by the complex perceptual and intellectual disabilities, and their interaction with physical problems, are those given by *Adams and Hurwitz* in a series of publications – for example, in 1963.

Depression is extremely common after strokes, including those due to subarachnoid haemorrhage. For example, *Murrell* et al. [1983] studied a representative population sample of 962 men and 1,555 women aged 55 years and over in Kentucky, using a standardised depression scale. Of women who had strokes 64% were depressed, compared to 16% of women without strokes; and the equivalent figures for men were 43 and 13%. Other studies have shown similar very high rates – higher than those with other severely disabling diseases.

Goodstein [1983] takes a broad view of the physical, mental and social problems of stroke survivors. He points out that 70% of them are vocationally impaired, and that one-third are totally dependent on their families or other help. He lists and comments on many of the problems the patients have: the humiliation of incontinence or of messy feeding, the loss of dignity and self-esteem, the awareness of changed appearance and impaired sexuality, the catastrophic reactions to tasks of daily living, and many others. He also discusses the reactions of the family, and emphasizes the value of discussion and education for the family, pointing out that for those in institutions the staff are the family, in a way.

In the series of 261 SAH patients followed up by *Storey* [1972], about one-quarter were rated as depressed. In those with aneurysms the presence of brain damage correlated highly with depression, but in the small group with normal angiograms, with almost no residual brain damage, there was also high rates of depression. As mentioned earlier, that subgroup had vulnerable personalities with a high rate of psychiatric morbidity before the bleed, being prone to anxiety, reserved rather than outgoing, and lacking in 'energy'.

Depression in the aneurysm cases was most common in those with posterior communicating aneurysms, which are closely related to the hypothalamus, and there is perhaps a causal relationship in that connection.

The role of personality factors in depression after subarachnoid haemorrhage from aneurysm was interesting: depression was significantly commoner in those brain damaged who were regarded as more 'energetic' in their daily lives before the SAH, unlike those without aneurysms. It seemed that those who had put most into living suffered the greatest 'loss' from their disabilities.

Most of the many studies published consider the emotional state of the stroke survivor in terms of an understandable reaction to the suffering they endure and the problems they face. We are all aware, of course, that many patients show no depressive change and can instead be fatuously cheerful or 'denying'. Another approach to this attempts to link emotional state to site of damage in ways which are not simply empathic. The subject of cerebral laterality and psychopathology is reviewed by *Gruzelier* [1981], who concludes that there is good evidence linking right hemisphere dysfunction to depressive states, and left-sided dysfunction to manic states, although the latter is less well supported, and there are 'contradictory findings'. *Gruzelier's* review, however, is not concerned with stroke illnesses as such, but more with psychophysiological studies in depressives.

Robinson and his colleagues, in a series of publications [e.g. *Robinson* et al., 1984], claim that strokes with left anterior cerebral damage are more likely to lead to depression, and the more anterior the lesions the more severe the depression. Right anterior lesions, they claim, lead to a cheerful and apathetic frame of mind; but right hemisphere lesions are likely to lead to depression when they are more posterior. (When, of course, they are more likely to have the visuospatial and body image disorders which are so troublesome and 'depressing' in an understandable way, as described by many others.)

Another approach is that of *Ross and Rush* [1981], who think that damage to the right anterior brain leads to a loss of the ability to describe emotions, whereas right posterior lesions lead to a loss of the recognition of feelings: analogous to the expressive and receptive dysphasias which characterise anterior and posterior lesions of the left hemisphere. Whether or not these cerebral localisation findings will stand up to replication studies remains to be seen, but they are important in trying to understand the complex and, at times, paradoxical-seeming results of strokes.

Conclusion

Stroke illnesses are one of the most important causes of death and disability. Hypertension is the principal antecedent, and psychosomatic interest in the causes of strokes must be focussed on the causes of hypertension. So far, the evidence linking high blood pressure and emotional factors is not impressive, although there are some interesting leads. Other factors in the genesis of strokes, such as diet and exercise, have obvious psychosocial aspects in the broad sense, even if there is no apparent direct role for emotional and personality influences at present. Strokes can be finally precipitated by major emotional upheaval, as has long been known, but this is presumably in those already predisposed by hypertension and atherosclerosis. Subarachnoid haemorrhage in patients with normal angiograms is relatively uncommon and relatively non-serious, but has the interesting distinction apparently of being more directly linked to emotional and personality factors than any other form of cerebrovascular accident.

Strokes lead to great suffering and disability, and study of the survivors throws light not only on the emotional reactions of individuals to varying severe forms of stress and loss, but also on some functions of the brain, and on the localisation of those functions.

References

Adams, G.F.; Hurwitz, L.J.: Mental barriers to recovery from strokes. Lancet *ii:* 533–537 (1963).
Adler, R.; MacRitchie, K.; Engel, G.L.: Psychologic processes and ischemic stroke (occlusive cerebrovascular disease). I. Observations on 32 men with 35 strokes. Psychosom. Med. *33:* 1–29 (1971).
Benton, A.L.: Behavioural change in cerebrovascular disease (Harper & Row, New York 1970).
British Medical Journal: Leader. Symptoms in hypertension. Br. med. J. *i:* 1551–1552 (1976).
Carasso, R.; Yehuda, S.; Ben-Uriah, Y.: Personality type, life events, and sudden cerebrovascular attack. Int. J. Neurosci. *14:* 223–225 (1981).
Cobb, S.; Rose, R.M.: Hypertension, peptic ulcer, and diabetes in air traffic controllers. J. Am. med. Ass. *224:* 489–492 (1973).

Cochrane, E.R.: Neuroticism and discovery of high blood pressure. J. psychosom. Res. *13:* 21–23 (1969).

D'Atri, D.A.; Fitzgerald, E.F.; Kasl, S.V.; Ostfield, A.M.: Crowding in prisons: the relationship between changes in housing mode and blood pressure. J. psychosom. Med. *43:* 95–106 (1981).

Ecker, A.: Emotional Stress before strokes. A preliminary report of 20 cases. Ann. intern. Med. *40:* 49–56 (1954).

Engel, G.L.: A psychological setting of somatic disease: the giving up-given up complex. Proc. R. Soc. Med. *60:* 553–555 (1967).

Foulds, G.: Personality and personal illness (Tavistock, London 1965).

Friedman, M.; Rosenman, R.H.: Association of specific overt behaviour patterns with blood and cardiovascular findings. J. Am. med. Ass. *169:* 1286–1296 (1959).

Gianturco, D.; Breslin, M.; Heyman. A.; Gentry, W.; Jenkins, C.; Kaplan, B.: Personality patterns and life stress in ischaemic cerebral vascular disease. Stroke *5:* 453–460 (1974).

Goldberg, D.P.: The detection of psychiatric illness by questionnaire. Maudsley Monogr. No. 22 (Oxford University Press, Oxford 1972).

Goodstein, R.K.: Overview: Cerebrovascular accident and the hospitalised elderly – a multidimensional clinical problem. Am. J. Psychiat. *140:* 141–147 (1983).

Gruzelier, J.H.: Cerebral laterality and psychopathology: fact and fiction. Psychol. Med. *11:* 219–227 (1981).

Heine, B.: Psychogenesis of hypertension Proc. R. Soc. Med. *63:* 1267–1280 (1970).

Henry, J.P.; Cassel, J.C.: Psychosocial factors in essential hypertension. Am. J. Epidem. *90:* 171–200 (1969).

Heyden, S · Stress im Arteriosklerosegeschehen. 2. Zerebrale Arteriosklerose und Apoplexie. Internist *19:* 642–648 (1978).

Holbrook, M.: Stroke: social and emotional outcome. J. R. Coll. Physns., Lond. *16:* 100–104 (1982).

Holmes, T.H.; Rahe, R.H.: The Social Readjustment Rating Scale. J. psychosom. Res. *11:* 213–218 (1967).

Kannel, W.B.: In Ross-Russell, Cerebral arterial disease (Churchill Livingstone, Edinburgh 1983).

Kidson, M.A.: Personality and hypertension. J. psychosom. Res. *17:* 35–42 (1973).

Lancet: Binge drinking and stroke (Editorial). Lancet *ii:* 660–661 (1983).

Leonberg, S.C.; Elliott, F.A.: Prevention of recurrent stroke. Stroke *12:* 731–735 (1981).

Lidell, J.A.: Review of book by John A. Lidell. A treatise on apoplexy, cerebral haemorrhage, cerebral embolism, cerebral gout, cerebral rheumatism and epidemic cerebrospinal meningitis (Wood, New York 1873); in Lancet, pp. 910–911.

Mann, A.: Hypertension: psychological aspects and diagnostic impact in a clinical trial. Psychol. Med. Monogr., suppl. 5 (Cambridge University Press, Cambridge 1984).

Marmot, M.: Culture and illness. Epidemiological evidence; in Christie, Mellett, Foundations of psychosomatics (Wiley, Chichester 1981).

Monk, M.: Psychologic status and hypertension. Am. J. Epidem. *112:* 201–207 (1980).

Murphy, E.; Brown, G.W.: Life events, psychiatric disturbance and physical illness. Br. J. Psychiat. *136:* 326–338 (1980).

Murrell, S.A.; Himmelfarb, S.; Wright, K.: Prevalence of depression and its correlates in older adults. Am. J. Epidem. *117:* 173–185 (1983).

Nefzeger, M.D.: Follow up studies of World War II and Korean War prisoners. Am. J. epidem. *91:* 123–138 (1970).
Parkes, C.M.; Benjamin, B.; Fitzgerald, R.G.: Broken heart. A statistical study of increased mortality among widowers. Br. med. J. *i:* 740–743 (1969).
Patel, C.; Marmot, M.G.; Terry, D.J.: Controlled trial of biofeedback aided behavioural methods in reducing mild hypertension. Br. med. J. *282:* 2005–2007 (1981).
Penrose, R.; Storey, P.: Emotional disturbance and sub-arachnoid haemorrhage. Psychother. Psychosom. *18:* 321–325 (1970).
Ritchie, D.: Stroke (Faber & Faber, London 1960).
Robinson, R.G.; Kudos, K.L.; Starr, L.B.; Rao, K.; Price, T.R.: Mood disorders in strokes. Importance of localisation of lesion. Brain *107:* 81–94 (1984).
Rosenman, R.H.; Friedman, M.; Strauss, R.; Wurm, M.; Jenkins, D.; Messinger, H.B.: Coronary heart disease in the western collaborative study. J. Am. med. Ass. *195:* 86–92 (1966).
Ross, E.D.; Rush, A.J.: Diagnosis and neuro-anatomical correlates of depression in brain damaged patients. Archs. gen. Psychiat. *38:* 1344–1354 (1981).
Sainsbury, P.: Neuroticism and hypertension in an outpatient population. J. psychosom. Res. *8:* 235–238 (1964).
Salonen, J.T.; Puska, P.; Tuomilehto: Physical activity and risk of myocardial infarction. cerebral stroke and death. Am. J. Epidemiol. *115:* 526–537 (1982).
Schmale, A.H.: A relationship of separation and depression to disease. Psychosom. Med. *20:* 259–277 (1958).
Seidenberg, R.; Ecker, A.: Psychodynamic and arteriographic studies of acute cerebral vascular disorders. Psychosom. Med. *16:* 374–392 (1954).
Sims, A.: Mortality in neurosis. Lancet *ii:* 1072–1075 (1973).
Sims, A.; Prior, P.: The pattern of mortality in severe neuroses. Br. J. Psychiat. *133:* 299–305 (1978).
Storey, P.B.: The precipitation of sub-arachnoid haemorrhage. J. psychosom. Res. *13:* 175–182 (1969).
Storey, P.: Emotional disturbances before and after sub-arachnoid haemorrhage; in Physiology, emotion and psychosomatic illness (Elsevier-Excerpta Medica, Amsterdam 1972).
Wadden, T.A.: Relaxation therapy for essential hypertension. Specific or non-specific effects? J. psychosom. Res. *28:* 53–61 (1984).

Peter Storey, MD, St. George's and Springfield Hospitals, London SW17 ORE (UK)

5. Psychosomatic Aspects of Multiple Sclerosis

J.W. Paulley

Lately Physician to the Ipswich Hospitals, Ipswich, Suffolk, UK

Multiple Sclerosis and Its Relationship to Psychiatric States

The literature on this topic is extensive and still growing. It has been reviewed on a number of occasions, *Cottrell and Wilson*, [1926], *Pratt* [1951], *Sai-Halasz* [1956], *Surridge* [1969], *Davison and Bagley* [1969] and *Trimble and Grant* [1983], to mention but a few. These reviews contain key references certainly until 1981 and it is therefore unnecessary to quote them again. However, a computerised search has recorded the following articles which may have escaped previous reviews, or which have been pusblished since. These are on mania [*Morton and Bonnefous*, 1976; *Kemp* et al. 1977; *Monaco* et al., 1980; *Mapelli* et al., 1981; *Peselow* et al., 1981], schizophrenia [*Payk*, 1983; *Matthews*, 1979; *Hollender and Steckler* 1972; *Salguero* et al., 1969], hysteria [*Caplan and Nadelson*, 1980], depression [*Lemere*, 1966; *Wender and Dominik*, 1972; *Caliezi*, 1981] and pseudoneurasthenic syndrome found by *Osuch* [1974] in 8.79% of 853 patients over 12 years. He considered its relationship to organic disease 'neglible'. Two other series are large and justify attention. 773 patients were studied during 1965–1971 by *Payk* [1973] and 50% showed some change in affect; only 5 had paranoid hallucinating psychosis. The other, by *Bulandra and Siferescu* [1968], of 178 patients, 14.6% of which showed what could be termed 'syndrome shift' with alternating physical and neurological symptoms. Uncertainty persists as to whether the variety of psychiatric disturbance, closely related in time to onset or relapse of multiple sclerosis (MS), is attributable to brain damage or not. The psychiatric disturbances reported since *Charcot's* [1877] observation have ranged widely from mood states, such as euphoria and belle indifférence, to hysteria and affective disorder (anxiety-depression) to the more rare but more dramatic psychotic episodes of mania, manic depressive psychosis and schizophrenia.

There have been important systematic studies in which the incidence of psychotic depression, mania and schizophrenia in large groups of multiple sclerosis patients have been compared with control groups. For the most part these studies have shown no significantly greater incidence in MS groups. On the other hand, the mood states of euphoria, belle indifférence, and denial, while frequently reported in MS patients have rarely been systemetically measured against controls. *Surridge's* [1969] study was exceptional. The mood states have also been considered by some [*Sai-Halasz,* 1956; *Runge,* 1928], including the author, to be premorbid (see premorbid patterns of behaviour, part II). The same in general applies to hysteria, but as *Trimble and Grant* [1983] and *Caplan and Nadelson* [1980] have pointed out, hysteria is an 'imprecise term', presenting many facets some of which will impress one observer but not the other. This may account for differing reports of its incidence in MS.

On balance, anxiety and depression have been found more frequently in MS patients than controls, and *Whitlock and Siskind* [1980] found that MS patients were more depressed than those controls who were also depressed, and that more MS patients also had had episodes of depression before the onset of neurological symptoms. In previous communications, *Paulley* [1976–77, 1977] described the tendency of all patients with MS to hide their emotions behind a smiling mask suggestive of euphoria or belle indifférence, while others hide behind a flat or unsmiling mask, which might be interpreted by some as depressive. This, therefore, could account for the widely differing reports on the incidence of depression as well as hysteria. *Charcot* [1877] described the unsmiling mask clearly: 'The look is vague and uncertain, the lips are hanging and half open, the features have a stolid expression...' and went on to report it as a 'state of mental depression'. However, the author prefers to see these 'mood states' as characteristics of these patients' shared poverty of emotional expression or denial, because longer acquaintance with them reveals that they are neither truly euphoric nor depressed, but are just covering up their feelings. It is rare for them to weep for more than a few seconds, then almost at once a single tear is replaced by a smiling face as if to repair the crack in the emotional defence they have always needed to cover their vulnerable inner core.

50 years ago organic brain disturbance seemed the most likely cause of the wide variety of psychiatric states in MS. That is understandable, and most doctors by their selection and training seek a tidy solution to a problem, rather than an untidy one. They prefer a hypothesis based on straight cause and effect rather than the possibility that observed effect and hypothesised cause are due to a common unsuspected provocative factor. The writer thinks that the very breadth of the spectrum of both psychiatric states and behaviour patterns in MS in itself favours this kind of explanation and can quote many clinical examples of this tandem phenomenon.

Freud [1923–1925] in his papers on ego psychology considered that characterological defences, such as hysterical, obsessional and depressive were archaic, instinctual and inherited, and that any individual could be expected to use one of these to reduce intense internal tension and anxiety arising from a severe emotional threat.

In the second part of this chapter the author will put forward evidence that a 'typical' form of emotional stress in definitively predisposed individuals is the major determinant in the pathogenesis of onset and relapse of MS. It is suggested, therefore, that both the wide variety of psychiatric states reported, and the somatic response leading to demyelination are *both the result of the same emotional threat,* thereby accounting for the close time relationship. The threat, in the majority of cases being unconscious or scarcely perceived, is related by only a minority to their physical or mental condition. Most people developing a severe visual disturbance or weakness of a limb are normally anxious or depressed, but as many reports testify, the psychiatric state may develop when the MS symptoms are so slight as to be barely recognisable by the patient. However, the frequency which MS patients use the hysterical defence and/or belle indifférence-denial was noted by *Charcot* and many others since. Many MS patients early in the illness, but with alarming symptoms, such as blindness, paraplegia and loss of bladder control give their history smiling, laughing, and making jokes in a most inappropriate manner. Later, when they or their relatives are asked whether this is usual for them to respond to alarming events in this way one learns that they have *always* concealed their emotions, even to the extent of laughing instead of crying when a friend at school broke a leg or was killed. In other words, evidence obtained from relatives, friends and patients points to inappropriate affect antedating their disease by many years and is inseparable from premorbid childlike behaviour, emotional immaturity and the giving-up response reported so frequently [*Charcot;* 1877; *Langworthy,* 1947; *Grinker* et al., 1950; *Mey-*

Tal et al, 1969; *Harrower,* 1950; *Philippopoulos* et al., 1958; *Paulley,* 1977].

A number of investigators have noted that patients with various psychosomatic disorders have had previous episodes of mental illness more often than anticipated when compared with controls. For example, *Goldberg* [1970] found this in his series of Crohn's disease. The phenomenon of sudden syndrome shift from ulcerative colitis to schizophrenia has been noted by the author, and also syndrome shift from asthma to an intense anxiety state or psychotic depression without a wheeze audible anywhere. This may occur spontaneously or during treatment.

However, patients with psychosomatic disorders, who have in common the difficulty in expressing, or even feeling, some emotions, tend to stay with the somatic pathway as a means of emotional expression. It seems once that avenue has been opened up it is subsequently preferred. Therefore, syndrome shift for them occurs more commonly from one psychosomatic disorder to another rather than to psychoneurosis or psychosis. Both *Arnason* [1975] and *Paulley* [1981] have a number of patients who have ulcerative colitis and MS with the former usually preceding MS. Probable reasons for this cross-association will be discussed in the next section.

It is not the author's brief to discuss the effect of, or frequency of, organic brain damage from demyelination on memory, cognitive function, onset of epilepsy or dementia. For an up-to-date review of this the reader is referred to *Trimble and Grant* [1983]. However, it is the author's experience that, as with other dementing disorders leading to cortical atrophy, such as GPI, cerebral arteriosclerosis, and pseudo-bulbar palsy, the patient's normal premorbid mood becomes exaggerated and a caricature of his or her normal mood. The exception being atypical and unexpected outbursts of violence, sometimes accompanied by a beatific smile to the great distress of close relatives, wholly unaware that patients with MS, normally so docile, have a great deal of pent up anger and resentment against frustrating key figures dating from childhood. It is the misfortune of surrogates to take the brunt of this release phenomenon.

Multiple Sclerosis as a Psychosomatic Disorder

The author considers that emotional stress is a major determinant in the causation of MS. This is based on his own experience and that of others quoted in a previous communication [*Paulley*, 1976] and confirmed by all 58 new cases he has seen since. This does not imply that other determinants are not involved, such as histocompatibility antigens (HLA) or other inherited disposition; nor *does it exclude* varying immunological responsiveness to a virus of widespread distribution. Epidemiological evidence appears to be against, rather than for a specific infective agent.

Vulnerability and 'Separation-Engulfment' Threats

The scene is set for both onset or relapse of MS when a characteristically vulnerable individual meets two quite specific forms of threat. The vulnerability is due to a failure to separate emotionally from parents or surrogates. The first of the threats is that of potential or actual emotional severance, but not necessarily involving physical separation, e.g. by marriage or emigration. Emotional threats commonly met with are illness or ageing of the key figure, or alienation leading to possible or actual withdrawal by the key figure. Inevitably, the primary key figure is the mother, but early surrogates may be father, a sibling or a grandparent. Some patients with MS succeed in overcoming losses of such key figures providing they find an adequate surrogate such as a spouse, and because the latter may be less frustrating in maintenance of the original bond a degree of separation may occur permitting a degree of emotional growth and independence. It follows, therefore, that the onset of MS may be deferred until a separation (or engulfment) threat develops between the patient and a surrogate, such as the spouse and/or the children of the marriage some of whom may have also become surrogates.

The second threat is that of emotional engulfment. *Mei-Tal* et al. [1969] noted the same factor, but called it 'entrapment'. This may seem paradoxical in view of what has been said about separation, but of which entrapment/engulfment is just the other side of the coin. Some readers may require a brief explanation. Within every living being there is the biological necessity of attaining independent existence of the parent. It is longest in the primates, with chimpanzees needing 5–7 years to attain maturity and in man 15–20 years, according to the culture. It is common knowledge, however, that biological independence is not always accompanied by emotional independence. In man, emotional development progresses from infancy through childhood until the end of adolescence. *Freud*

[1924] and *Erikson* [1959] have identified important stages in that development, none more important than that which occurs when the infant, having been wholly dependent on its mother for its very existence, begins to see itself as 'me' and 'not part of you'. Some workers such as *Klein* [1932] have maintained that this process starts immediately after birth, but to the ordinary observer it becomes apparent between 6 months and 3 years with the physical independence of locomotion, feeding, of control of bladder and bowel, and necessary assertion of the toddler's emotional independence often expressed in negativism to commands and requests by the parent. Patients with MS recall degrees of failure to establish this first stage of independence and for a wide variety of reasons. 'I could never cross my mother' they may say. It will only be possible here to give a few examples, such as a mother near her menopause maintaining the stage of infantile dependence by her child beyond infancy to satisfy her own emotional need. The same may occur with long-awaited only children. Such patients may speak of their childhood environment as cosy like a cocoon, but for all that as restrictive as a steel cage. Other patients may tell how they had to go to relatives because their mother was admitted to hospital shortly after their birth and of their consequent fear of losing her again leaving them clinging, obedient and docile. Such children fear to rock the frail boat of their security by the most trival push towards independence, such as by not going to bed when asked, or refusing to put their boots on. Another reason for not attaining emotional independence is that they are terrified of excessive emotional response on the part of the key figure, either of rage or extreme displays of anxiety or tears, particularly when a sibling or the patient displeases. Some patients remember a brother being beaten for a minor misdemeanour or assertion of independence and thereby learn that they should not risk it themselves.

At the second important stage of development at puberty, the child in effect is saying 'I am no longer a child, I am now an adult'. Once again MS patients describe great difficulties in surmounting this hurdle, indeed, the author has yet to meet one who has achieved it although they may claim to have done so by confusing physical distance with emotional distance. The cocooned child fails because it fears the separation threat of a hurt parent withdrawing emotionally, while the tyranised child recalls efforts to do so being put down by penalties or threats of withdrawal by the key figure. Finding the way barred by both types of response, they sometimes make what is for them an outrageous rebellion, such as suddenly leaving home, throwing up a chosen career, becoming pregnant, etc. However, these vulnerable people are in the constant emotional dilemma of wanting to be 'out' when they are 'in', yet when they achieve a modest degree of 'outness' they feel they must be 'in', again in case their temerity should have permanently *impaired* the almost placental relationship without which they suffer feelings of horror only comparable to that of an abandoned infant, i.e. for survival itself.

Separation-Engulfment in Terms of Behaviourist or Life Event Theory

The giving-up response in the face of these threats (stimuli) can also be looked at in terms of learning theory and conditioning. In childhood the 'giving-up' response to threats of separation or engulfment is 'rewarded' by reduction of the resultant tension and a return to physiological homeostasis. However, the adolescent or adult finds the giving-up response less and less effective in assuaging tension arising from these stimuli. This is in part because they are chronologically no longer children, and because separation previously only threatened becomes more and more of a reality with ageing, sick, dying or alienated key figures. At the same time 'engulfment', tolerated in childhood, becomes less and less acceptable as previously unconscious feelings rise near to consciousness and the individual discovers that he lacks any alternative coping mechanism other than 'giving-up' (this also happens in adolescence in ulcerative colitis and Crohn's disease). Tension therefore persists following each stimulus, indeed successive failures to 'win' against threats of engulfment or separation seem only to 'reinforce' the patient's long conditioning to feel helpless, hopeless and to give up. The extreme sensitivity of MS patients to events most people might feel as trivial, or irrelevant, of which examples will be given and which increases with age, suggests that 'reinforcement' may be instrumental in intensifying such sensitivity. On the other hand, apparently spontaneous and lengthy remissions in MS could be regarded as due to a degree of deconditioning as much as any lessening of previously intolerable external events. Thus, periods of relative security and tranquility might allow such a degree of 'deconditioning' to occur [see 'girl of 16' top of p. 33 *Paulley,* 1976].

Similarly, 'life event' theorists can also be acommodated if they can stretch their concept to include a long adverse and running relationship of the child with its parents and other key figures as an 'event' or as summation of minor events.

Childlike Dependency

As mentioned in the section of psychiatric states in MS these sensitive people often seem childlike or young for their age, and use defences to cover tenderness such as the masks, belle indifférence, and denial. Many observers have commented on childlike behaviour, the first being *Charcot* [1877] who used the term 'puerilisme mentale'; *Langworthy* [1947] also noted 'emotional immaturity' and 'an entangling neurotic relationship with the mother'. *Grinker* et al., [1950] wrote 'the premorbid state of the multiple sclerotic is that of great immaturity since early infancy', and *Mei-Tal* et al., [1969] 'Interpersonal relationships are characterised by strong dependence needs'. *Harrower* [1950] reported 'a high incidence of passive dependency', and *Philippopoulos* et al., [1958] 'emotional and psychosexual immaturity'. *Paulley* [1976–77] noted a pathological dependence on a parental key figure transferred wholly or partly to other key figures.

Life Events Research

Studies have confirmed that more patients with multiple sclerosis than controls suffer threatening significant life event threats prior to the onset of or relapses of their disease [*Pratt*, 1951; *Mei-Tal et al., 1970; Grant*, this vol.]. *Warren* et al., [1982] in a study of 100 patients with 100 hospital case controls, found that significantly more MS patients had suffered significant 'life-event' stress in the previous 2 years according to *Brown's* [1974] criteria. Such information can be obtained in a normal medical history in approximately 30% of patients providing the interviewer is empathetic and affords enough time. However, only recently has this form of research recognised the importance of the meaning of or impact of a particular life event to the individual and tried to rate it. *Brown* [1974], *Mei-Tal* et al., [1969] and *Paulley* [1976–77, 1983] stressed that a life event in itself meant little without assessment of its intrapsychic meaning to the patient. Attention was drawn to the same point following the Empire Rheumatism Council's negative report on Stress in Relation to Rheumatoid Arthritis in 1950 [*Paulley* 1950]. However, it has to be said that unless 'facilitating' techniques of the type described in this chapter are used in future, life event researchers will continue to underscore.

Psychosomatic Aspects of Multiple Sclerosis

Identifying the Provocative Life Event and Its Intrapsychic Meaning: The First Essential

To do this the doctor or therapist needs to return time and time again to the question ' what did you *actually feel* when this happened?' Patients reply eventually with such terms as 'horror', 'cold', 'frozen', 'empty', 'hopeless', 'helpless', 'defeated' ('defighted' said one) and these may be accompanied by a deep sigh epitomising the giving-up response.

Because the precipitant life event is not in the patient's consciousness in approximately 70% of cases, facilitating techniques of interviewing or the help of spouses, siblings and fiancé(e)s are required to identify it. This cannot be emphasised too strongly because the first essential in psychotherapy for these patients is to identify with them the provocative stress as early as possible after the first attack or a relapse. The author has made the same point in the psychological management of ulcerative colitis and Crohn's disease [*Paulley,* 1981]. Some physicians and neurologists may think that discovering a provocative event not perceived consciously by the patient will be too difficult. In reality it is not, given a little patience and above all the knowledge of where to look. Indeed, what gardener digs for potatoes in the rose garden?

At the first consultation, when a diagnosis of MS seems probable, although unconfirmed, it is useful to ask 'would you be surprised if this trouble you have with your eye, and your weak leg six months ago, might have been provoked by emotional stress'. The author's experience is that 50% of cases reply that they 'would not be surprised' and in the 50% replying negatively a spouse or partner 'will not be surprised' when they are seen together, especially if the pump is primed by giving examples of typically provocative separation-engulfment life events from other patients' histories.

Some Examples

A woman of 30, whose husband said she and her mother were like sisters and never apart, presented with retrobulbar neuritis and was asked if she had had any shocks or bad news prior to the attack. At first she could not think of any, but after being given a few examples the interview proceeded:

(Patient) P: 'I know I listen to the neighbour, she has just lost her father'. (Doctor) D: 'Has she?' P: 'Mmm, I suppose it sort of makes you think sometimes, you know, it could happen to my father'. D: 'I know, when did it happen? How long ago?' P: 'Last week, last Wednesday, I think he died.' D: 'But you felt all that in your bones?' (Pause) P: 'Well, I kept imagining it was my father, you know what I mean.' D: ('rewarding' patient by shaking hands) 'I think you did.' P: 'I often do, and think what would you do then, you know, I run off and do all things like that'. D: 'You began to get inside the other woman's shoes?' P: 'Most probably'. D: 'You don't remember which day you heard about it?' P: 'Well he had been ill for about a fortnight, he was in hospital, I think it was last Wednesday he died'. D: 'that was 1–2 days before your eye trouble. Do you remember what you *felt* when the news was broken?' P: 'Mmm, well I felt a little bit sad I felt, as you say unconsciously it was my father and that, but seeing he is an older man – although (hurriedly) he is very well and that he is not feeling ill or anything'. D: 'Surely.' P: 'I've always been fairly close to him as far back as I can remember'. D: 'Yes.' P: 'I always got on well with him.' D: 'I understand.'

Another woman had a relapse when the next door neighbour's mother dropped dead, again the woman was approximately the same age as her own mother, and in both these cases the deceased stood for the patient's parents while the patient identified with the bereaved daughters.

A Useful Question

A useful 'tin-opening' question in interviewing these vulnerable people is to ask them 'how they feel about "goodbyes"?' Universally, they say goodbyes greatly distress them. They can then be asked to explain why, and when they have experienced it, and how their parents or surrogates reacted.

A vulnerable woman had lost one eye as a result of falling on some scissors while playing with her father in the garden when she was 2. Her close attachment to him dated from then. Several admissions to hospital followed, and at the age of 5 the damaged eye was removed. She had never been able to win her mother's approval or go against her and thought that this was because of her mother's jealousy of her relationship with her father. Shortly after the onset of MS aged 28, her husband, giving an example of her sensitivity, said that during courtship she had always been in tears if any distance away from home. However, marriage brought a degree of independence for the first time. Her MS began aged 28 when unconsciously ambivalent about having a baby, a decision which could not be deferred much longer. She felt threatened because all her friends were having babies and by the knowledge that her husband wanted one. (Approximately 25% of patients with MS have a 'hang-up' over babies which will be discussed in detail later.) The woman in question after several joint interviews recognised her unconscious ambivalence and made a conscious decision not to have a baby. Instead, a large black cat became her child. The significance of this became apparent when she came up one day saying that she had a relapse the day before. D: 'Perhaps this had something to do with your appointment?' Her husband nodded agreement. D: 'What was in your mind?' P: 'I feared you might keep me in hospital.' D: 'Why would you find that so frightening – I have never suggested it.' P: 'Because it would take me away from my husband (hesitation) my home' – long hesitation. D: 'And?' P: 'My cat'. A combination of an anticipated separation from her cat, and engulfment (entrapment) by her doctor.

The following is another example of the need to pursue the intrapsychic meaning of a life event.

A woman had her first attack of MS in December and the only thing that she could think of that had disturbed her shortly prior to this was hearing that her daughter of 13 was going to France with the school in the following April. She did not know why this had made her panic, but acknowledged that it would be the first time that her daughter would be away from her. Later she revealed she had forbidden the trip the previous year, saying her daughter was too young. Possible reasons for her feelings were explored but with negative results. Only after four interviews, and asked once again to recall what she *actually felt* on receiving the letter from the school, was she able to speak of a terrifying fantasy in which her daughter was on the top deck of the boat crossing the Channel in a rough sea and falling overboard. She then recalled her own first Channel crossing at the age of 8 in a very rough sea.

Another woman of 45, widowed for 9 years with a married daughter developed her first episode 2 days after hearing that the daughter's husband was moving to another part of the country. After her husband's death her daughter and grandchildren had become surrogates, and she visited them every weekend; she had no other relative. For 6 months and several interviews she was unable to describe her feelings on hearing the news using denial and rationalisation as defences. Then one day, asked once again what she had actually felt when her daughter told her, she replied 'Horror'. D: 'Thats a very strong word.' P: 'Well that's what I felt ... everything seemed empty and hopeless.'

Yet another woman hiding her sensitivity behind the flat mask was unable to think of a provocative stress leading to her first attack, until her husband reminded her that it had occurred as she was walking across the Speedway Stadium where her younger son was about to race for the first time. In her imagination she felt he would be killed.

Similar threats of engulfment closely related in time to MS, some so overwhelming as to cause patient's to feel 'helpless' and 'hopeless' and 'defeated' remain in the patients unconscious until facilitating techniques in therapy help them to bring them into consciousness. The following are examples.

A woman, an only child, with very dominant parents achieved a measure of geographical but not emotional independence by using her intellect to qualify for a profession. One day, one of her superiors attacked her verbally in the way she had experienced in childhood, she felt 'put down' and unable to reply, an MS episode followed 2 days later. Another MS episode occurred when her husband had been unfairly and publicly criticised by a colleague; the patient felt for her husband as if it had been herself.

Another patient with MS learned that her husband had been sacked unfairly by his employer and had a relapse of MS her first attack having occurred 6 years previously when she suddenly became ataxic walking up a hill to a hospital where her only son was having an emergency nephrectomy. She said she was not worried about her husband because he was highly qualified and able to get a new job. So what had upset her? 'It was the nasty way it was done and his employer is a little man.' Asked what that had to do with it, she said ' all little men are like that, my father was a little man and he terrified my mother and all of us'. Here was clear identification with her husband being put down by another ' little man' who stood in her thoughts for her tyrannical father. Indeed, her father had a tantrum on her wedding day and tried to stop her leaving the house.

MS patients conceal their emotions behind a smiling or a flat unsmiling mask, as described in the previous communication [*Paulley,* 1976–77]. The cases quoted all hid behind the smiling mask and demonstrate that at one time the provocative threat may be engulfment and at another separation. It should not be forgotten that pets may also be surrogates. For example, a woman who went on holiday had for the first time to leave her dogs in kennels and had an attack because she could not stop thinking of them, or the fantasied fear of a cat returning to its old home and being killed crossing the main road. The cases also illustrate how the threats do not always involve the patient themselves, but only indirectly because of identification with some one in their immediate environment, not necessarily a relative, but who for some reason suddenly stands for a key figure. In other words they fear the threat of 'separation' or 'engulfment' 'second hand' by identification.

Marriage, Pregnancy, Childbirth and Babies

These are well recognised as potentially traumatic life events, along with redundancy, accidents, retirement and death, and it has long been acknowledged that some patients either develop MS, or relapse very closely in time relationship to pregnancy or childbirth. Not so well known is that the decision to have a baby may itself constitute the provocative threat in a susceptible individual. Many doctors and neurologists advise MS patients not to have children and sometimes to be sterilized. However, as mentioned previously [*Paulley,* 1976–77], it is not aways the woman who develops MS or relapses when a baby is born; fathers are also vulnerable to the threat of childbirth showing that pregnancy and parturition are not responsible. Nor is it uncommon for MS to occur or relapse when patients are not themselves involved in procreation but when their friends or siblings are having babies. Even to be asked to be a godparent or to attend a christening may be sufficient provocation. For example, *Mei-Tal* et al.

[1969] quote case No. 12 who developed an attack when her twin sister had a baby, and the author knows several cases where attacks occurred within hours or a day of either a christening or the birth of a baby to a sister or someone else. The event thus poses an intrapsychic threat through identification, because of the patient's ambivalence about having a child themselves [*Paulley*, 1977, p. 104]. *Inman* [1948], an eye surgeon and psychoanalyst, reported his findings in patients with MS over the previous 20 years and also noted the close temporal relationship to childbirth. He felt that sexual fantasies and guilt were involved. However, a long succession of patients have taught the author that the provocative threat is 'separation' posed by the baby to their own position as the dependent 'child' of their spouse. Patients with this problem may consciously want a baby, but unconsciously do not, and find all sorts of reasons to put it off.

A woman had felt cheated of her own childhood; she was 5 when she became 'little mother' to 4 younger brothers and sisters having until then been the spoilt younger child of the first family. At marriage she and her husband agreed that they would not have children. 'I had had enough of them' she said. She was 39 when her husband announced that he would like a boy because there was none in the family. She agreed but unfortunately it was a girl. Her first symptoms of MS occurred at a wedding when her daughter Jane was 18 months old. She told how, when the nappy stage had finished, her husband began to take Jane everywhere, 'he cared next to nothing for me, I felt left out, and have been left out ever since, and I am never consulted about anything'.

A very vulnerable and sensitive only son whose childlike attempts at independence were crushed by a mother who kept a cane, had clearly looked for some compensation for the bleakness of his own childhood when he married. Unfortunately, he was unsuccessful and he developed MS shortly after the birth of his first child. D: 'Did you have doubts about starting a family?' P: (long pause) 'No.' D: 'Were you keener or was your wife keener on starting a family?' P: 'My wife was keener.' D: 'And what did you say at the time, we haven't enough cash in the bank, or not been married long enough, or ...' P: 'No, no, I didn't express an opinion.' D: 'But you may have had reservations then?' P: 'I can't recall any.' D: 'No, but you had reservations as soon as the first child was born?' P: 'Yes.' D: 'You felt in the cold?' P: 'Yes.' D: 'It hit you?' P: 'It did – my wife said if you want affection now you'll have to find somebody else.' D: 'Do you remember what you felt?' P: (Long pause) 'I felt I did not know how she could do it to me' (giving up response).

Another woman with MS who had a relapse when her daughter was about to have her second child, when asked what she felt said 'sad'. Pressed at ensuing interviews to think why she had felt sad she said eventually 'poor Jason'. D: 'Why poor Jason?' P: 'Because he will be so hurt'. Jason was 6 and the first grandchild. The patient was identifying with Jason because both she and her sister, who also had MS, had been similarly displaced from their mother's affection by three younger brothers who followed.

For the sake of brevity the reader is referred to other examples, described in a previous communication [*Paulley*, 1976, cases 5 and 7], and also to *Barbellion's* [1948] autobiographical description of his response to the birth of his own baby quoted briefly by *Paulley* [1976] and discussed in the 'Summary'.

When a Doctor's Advice Can Be Damaging

Physicians' and neurologists' advice to MS patients not to have children, or to be sterilized, can be as dangerous for them as having a child, because without children, many fear, at least unconsciously, for the durability of their marriage. Some suffer terrifying fantasies of their spouse's infidelity even if he (or she) is out for an hour or two. It is, therefore, not uncommon for a patient to relapse within a day or two of the news of a relative's or close friend's marriage breaking up, or being made privy to some one else's infidelity. Suddenly, they see it as happening to them. Terrified, they suffer the 'giving up' response [*Mei-Tal* et al., 1969]. Usually, they identify with the injured spouse, but in therapy may reveal their identification to have been with one of the deserted children. For these reasons it is of great importance that MS patients should not be *just told* to avoid children or *told* that they should be sterilized without psychotherapeutic help to enable them to reach such a decision, as far as possible, free of unconscious 'hang-ups' over babies which affect as many as 25%. Clearly, to advise against having children in a patient who does not have this particular 'hang-up' is as unjustifiable as it is cruel. The author has seen many unfortunate women who deeply regret accepting such advice from doctors given in all good faith, but in ignorance of the consequences.

Psychological Management and/or Psychotherapy

Readers may well ask what can be done for these patients. Having elicited the particular stressful life event recalled by about 30% by standard history taking, yet perhaps only tentatively related by the patient to onset or relapse of MS, it is necessary to help them to uncover the intrapsychic impact of the event which is still unconscious. For the remaining 70%, where the precipitant life event has not been perceived, it can be made accessible using the kind of facilitating techniques already described and if 'typical' areas of provocation are explored ('the potato patch not the rose garden'). It is the author's experience, using psychodynamically orientated psychotherapy over the last 14 years, that approximately five out of ten patients can be helped materially, either going into long remissions, or by greatly reducing the number, severity and duration of their attacks. Another 2 out of 10 probably can be helped, leaving approximately 3 out of 10 who deteriorate despite attempts to help them with psychotherapy, ACTH, diets or any other means. Usually, the reasons for this are either lack of sufficient ego strength or because the domestic situation is so unfavourable or overwhelming that the patient has almost no chance of obtaining even the smallest degree of emotional independence (the 'Lorna Doone' syndrome) [*Paulley,* 1976]. Unfortunately, such patients are soon symbolically back to infancy, first toddling, and then back further in time to nappies and incontinence of bladder and bowel ('Psychophysiological regression') [*Philippopoulos* et al., 1958]. Therefore, an advanced state of disease itself inevitably creates physical dependence, but all too often accompanied by equivalent loss of any emotional independence which for MS sufferers has been so hard won. Thus, a vicious circle develops with relatives and care-givers 'engulfing' the patient with understandable anxiety, guilt and consequent over-concern. Such patients tend to deteriorate rapidly. The prognostic figures given are, of course, approximate and are offered only for guidance pending validation by a long-term trial which will require matched controls.

Assessment Suitability for
Psychotherapy and/or Psychological Management

From what has just been said, the cards are stacked against success for psychotherapy in the advanced case. Nevertheless, it may be possible to delay the ultimate deterioration, bowel and bladder incontinence. *Smith* [1975], such a case himself [cited by *Paulley,* 1976–77] described in a letter to *The Observer* his own flash of self-recognition and subsequent clinical improvement. The author is of the opinion that all patients early in their illness should be given the benefit of psychological management and/or psychotherapy. Assessment of likely success can usually be made after the first four interviews when one has gained some idea of the patient's ego strength, and the amount of help that is likely to be forthcoming from a 'co-therapist', i.e. husband, wife, partner, fiancé(e) or occasionally a sibling. When the factors mentioned are particularly adverse, psychotherapy fails like every other treatment for this disease has done to date. Thus, a few patients may receive a substantial amount of therapeutic time yet be dead within a year or two of the onset. These cases are as instructive as they are sad, but it does not require psychiatric experience for a physician or neurologist to recognise a hopeless prognosis when his patient faces the deadly combination of psychological inadequacy and very adverse environmental factors.

What Kind of Psychotherapy or Psychological Management?

Ruesch [1948] reported as long ago as 1948 that patients with psychosomatic disorders were unsuited to orthodox psychoanalytic methods. He wrote: 'In applying traditional methods of adult psychotherapy to treatment one discovers that these methods are unable to promote maturation ... The character is chronologically adult but emotionally a child.' Many psychoanalysts have since come to similar conclusions [*Marty and de M'Uzan*, 1963], while *Nemiah* [1972] noted their failure to move 'Despite months of intensive and persistent work. They come out of therapy as incapable of experiencing and describing affect and fantasy as when they entered it.' Thus, it is generally agreed that all psychosomatic patients share the common denominator of 'a poverty of emotional expression' and frustrate orthodox dynamic psychotherapists by their inability or reluctance to fantasise, free associate and present dreams. *Sifneos* [1973] summed it up 'these patients are not good candidates for dynamic psychotherapy'. *Wittich* [personal commun.] feels that a few can benefit from psychoanalysis but only after about 2 years of directive psychotherapy. Another reasonable objection by orthodox psychotherapists is that most patients suffering from psychosomatic disorders such as MS are too sick mentally to work with, i.e. able to tolerate or benefit from the standard therapeutic approach. Nevertheless, the increasing numbers of psychotherapists prepared to be more eclectic and more directive can be assured that MS patients, like so many other patients with psychosomatic disorders hitherto sadly neglected, await the deployment of their skills. Ideally, the therapist needs to feel secure enough to cope with patients' flights into the somatic expression of their underlying emotional problems, i.e. episodes of MS at the same time as helping them towards coping maturely with the threats of separation and engulfment. This means that a therapist with an adequate training in internal medicine has an advantage and suggests that a clinician may therefore be best placed to do this work providing he is equipped, or equips himself, with sufficient psychodynamic skills [*Aring,* 1965]. *Engel* [1958] also felt the same about the psychological management of ulcerative colitis, a disorder with a very comparable psychopathogenesis to MS.

Syndrome Shift

It is therefore not too surprising in view of what has just been said that the author has had 11 patients with ulcerative colitis and 1 with Crohn's disease who have also developed MS [*Paulley,* 1981]. Independently, *Arnason* [1975] also reported 7 such cases of MS and ulcerative colitis in 1975. On the other hand, syndrome shift from MS to other psychosomatic disorders with very different personality profiles and psychopathogenesis such as hypertension, asthma or the autoimmune diseases either does not occur or it is very rare. However, several MS patients seem to suffer from vasospastic conditions such as migraine or Raynaud's phenomenon, and a few have or have had idiopathic hirsuitism or anorexia nervosa.

Minimum Psychological Skills Needed for
Psychological Management of MS

(a) Knowledge of the stages of psychological development. (b) Mechanisms of identification. (c) Transference and counter-transference. (d) An understanding of methods of facilitation 'in pursuit of intrapsychic meanings of what appear to be trivial events in relation to separation and engulfment threats'. (e) An understanding of the paramount importance of spacing of interviews and of the mode of termination of psychotherapy or psychological management in which separation-engulfment threats are constantly involved in the transference and counter-transference, and by unconscious manipulation. Successful negotiation of this phase is perhaps the greatest contribution a therapist can make to a patient with this disorder in which separation and engulfment are basic to the psychopathogenesis. Thus, after the initial phase, the patient and not the therapist or doctor should decide the date of the next interview. With this kind of facilitation the patient comes to see the relationship of attacks and relapses to separation and engulfment threats and with the help of therapist and any 'co-therapist' such as a partner or spouse, learns to anticipate threats and may thereby succeed in forestalling them. The 'co-therapist' may be likened to a lightning conductor or a defuser of bombs! At the same time the patient learns to alter the ingrained coping response of 'giving up' and feeling 'hopeless', dating from childhood.

In the event of relapse, the patient and spouse (if available) need early access to the clinician or therapist so that the provocative emotional event, and its intrapsychic meaning, can be brought into consciousness where there is every chance of the patient being able to deal with it in an adult way. As has been said of ulcerative colitis and Crohn's disease [*Paulley* 1981], relapses need not be seen as disasters by the patient, or their relatives or doctor, providing the patient learns something from them, and are regarded as stepping stones to greater emotional maturity. As in all forms of this kind of work the patient must 'be held' long enough in the therapeutic relationship for psychological change to take place. With the extreme dependent vulnerability of patients suffering from disorders such as MS and ulcerative colitis, it is therefore necessary for the doctor or therapist for some months at least to be more supportive than is regarded as wise or in the patient's interest in the teachings of more orthodox psychotherapy. Without this, patients either drop out of therapy or relapse somatically (retreat into illness). However, the doctor must beware that 'support' is not seen by the patient as 'engulfment'.

One other caveat, patients always ask what the doctor feels about other forms of treatment such as the 'Russian vaccine' (happily dead!), diets, hyperbaric oxygen and spiritual healing. It is necessary if the doctor is not to 'engulf' or 'put down' his patient for him to say that he has no objection to any additional form of treatment the patient or his relatives wish to be pursued, provided it is not seen as an *alternative* but *additional* to the psychological work. Put another way, the patient must be helped to see that they will be tempted to seize on to dietetic or physical treatment in preference to psychological work which is harder and at times more painful. Without this kind of understanding the doctor or therapist will fail to 'hold' his patient, or the patient will pay only lip service without really 'working' just to keep his therapist happy and avoid the separation threat.

MS Associations and Societies

Most MS patients join such groups for the obvious reasons of obtaining help and information and the wish to support research. However, a few are fearful of attending meetings at which very disabled people may be present and seek their doctor's opinion about it. He should be careful. If he says 'No' he puts himself in the rôle of the engulfing parent as well as posing a separation threat if overconcerned relatives, friends, and usually a health visitor as well are pressing the patient to join. On the other hand, he should not say 'Yes' without first helping patients express their unconscious feelings about meeting dedicated organisers and 'engulfing' caregivers who tend to infantilize MS patients by doing too much for them or worst of all getting them into wheel chairs prematurely. Unfortunately, these are not rare experiences of some patients prevailed upon to go to camps or cruises before they are as disabled as their fellows with advanced disease for whom such events are truly the highlight of their monotonous lives. Lastly, patients themselves can be tactless and often tend to engulf 'the new boy or girl'. Doctors and care-givers need always to be aware of MS patients' sensivity and vulnerability to things which most people would not notice.

Duration of Psychological Management/Psychotherapy

Patients and relatives ask, when about to embark on psychological management and/or psychotherapy, how long they will need to attend and how frequently. The author has found, contrary to most teachings from orthodox psychotherapy, that the passage of time is probably more important to these patients' ability to change than the frequency of attendances or intensity of therapy. His reply therefore to the first question is, not less than 2 years and possibly 3–5 years, but by that time interviews may be spaced to 6 months, or even annually. Frequency of interviews initially will depend upon the severity of the case, and the patient's reactions at first interview. It is usually wise to see a patient not less than 3 weeks after the first interview and sometimes as little as a few days later if much psychological material has emerged, or there appears to be a need to hear a partner's feelings about the patient's alarming symptoms. The aim here is to give the partner (spouse) a positive rôle as a co-therapist rather than the one usually adopted for understandable reasons of being puzzled, frightened, guilty, and overconcerned, but all too much like an original engulfing parent and very counter-productive. For brevity, the reader is referred to the advantages of couple therapy in previous communications [*Paulley* [1976, 1977]].

A general practitioner, physician or neurologist before starting this kind of treatment will want to know how much time he may be letting himself in for. Ideally, he should allow for not less than half-an-hour per interview and preferably 1 h for the first. However, with the open access to outpatient clinics which the author recommends in the event of relapse, or a potentially threatening life situation, prior knowledge of the patient's problems enables much to be done in as little as 10 min. The first few months will involve the greatest expenditure of time, but by 6 months, interviews can often be spaced to 2–3 months. Some patients remit and then relapse after 3–4 years and require a further period of psychotherapy. For example, the author saw a patient recently whom he first saw in 1974 and who did well but relapsed again in 1978 when she thought she was pregnant with a third child. She had just obtained a good job, a most important step in her long and usually losing battle for independence. Once again she felt hopeless, trapped and unable to win. At her last attendance the patient was asked how many interviews she thought she had had over $9^{1}/_{2}$ years and answered 'about 20'. She was absolutely correct. Each interview would have varied between 10 min in an out-patient clinic to special sessions with her spouse varying between 30 and 45 min. Therefore, the total time for psychological management would have been approximately 10 h over $9^{1}/_{2}$ years which may be thought very moderate. The same amount of time would have been spent by many neurologists on some patients with MS in repeated neurological examinations, carrying out tests, and pursuing various treatments. After mutual agreement on termination, it is wise in this disorder for the therapist/doctor to assure the patient that his door will always be open if the patient feels the need to come back.

Is Psychological Management for MS Teachable or Must It Be Experiential?

It is the author's opinion that much of the technique can be described in words which is why he has risked boring his readers with more detail than is customary in articles or books dealing with treatment of other psychosomatic disorders. His belief is based on his own experience of going to Amsterdam 30 years ago when members of Prof. *Groen's* psychosomatic unit were able *to pass on to him* the skills that they had acquired in the psychological management of asthma. Prior to that, many of the author's asthmatic patients did badly and were frequently in need of re-admission, but subsequently management of asthma became a pleasure and a challenge to be overcome rather than the recurrent source of frustration and anxiety it had been before. However, as with any other technique, competence is only achieved by practice, and this is just as true for the psychological management of asthma or MS as it is for a surgical operation. Ideally, case management with some supervision by someone suitably trained would be worthwhile but at present there are few people able to do the supervision. Until there are, the author believes that videotape can be a great help in teaching and he has a large number of tapes illustrating progress of cases from presentation to termination, some extend over several years.

Research Possibilities

Lastly, we may consider what research possibilities offer for the validation or invalidation of the psychosomatic factor in pathogenesis. The author suggests that electro-magnetic tape (video) interviews provide an indelible record of an event as does an ECG or an EEG, and in the same way can be assessed and reassessed by independent observers. Controls interviewed and recorded in the same way could also be independently assessed for presence or absence of the particular features which the author and others such as *Mei-Tal* et al. [1969] and *Langworthy* [1947] have noted. Controls could suffer from other psychosomatic disorders, but not for example ulcerative colitis because emotional immaturity in that disease is very close to that of MS, and there is some syndrome shift between them. 'Healthy' controls would be better.

The other research that has yet to be done is a controlled study of the effectiveness of psychological management and/or psychotherapy against a control group. The author suggested such a trial 8 years ago with 50 patients and 50 matched controls to be studied over 5–7 years, their CNS state would have been assessed by an independent neurologist, and the study should have provided an indication as to whether the psychotherapy/psychological management group were doing better than the controls. It was assumed that both groups would receive standard methods of treatment including diets, hyperbaric oxygen, etc., and that the groups would be large enough to allow for treatment variations in each group to even out sufficiently for them to be discounted. Clearly, any attempted restriction on other forms of treatment that the controls or the patients might receive from their general practitioners, physicians, neurologists, homeopaths, herbalists, acupuncturists, etc., would be both unthinkable as well as unethical.

Research into the possible link between psyche and soma in MS, as in many other equally damaging disorders, need not wait elucidation of the somatic end of the chain of causation. Recent research suggests control of immunological competence via the limbic system and hypothalamus may be the link (see chapt. 1). Identification of an infective organism such as a virus would not invalidate the importance of an immunological determinant, herpes febrilis, provides a comparable model. There is one area of research which has received rather less attention over the last 30 years than before, and that is the vascular hypothesis for MS advanced by *Putnam* [1936]. Certainly, these patients are often vaso-spastic, and *Inman*, the eye surgeon and psychoanalyst, examining fundi, was struck by this, and in a personal communication urged the author not to neglect the possibility of a vascular link between psyche and soma.

A Summary of Earlier Psychosomatic Observations and Psychotherapeutic Work in MS and Conclusions

The first evidence of onset and relapse of MS fired by emotional threats of separation or engulfment in predisposed individuals was provided by sufferers from the disease. The first was *Augustus d'Este* 1794–1843 and the second *B.F. Cummings* 'Barbellion (pseudonym)', in the 'Journal of a disappointed man' [1948]. Their biographical accounts should be read by anyone wishing to understand the psychopathogenesis of MS. A few suitably selected and prepared patients can also benefit from the insight so gained, particularly from 'Barbellion's' sensitive account of his own vulnerability to the kind of threats already described in this chapter. On p. 287 he says: 'My pen is a delicate needle point tracing out a graph of temperament ... all my moods and vapours, all the varying reactions to environment of this jelly, which is I.' In the 1948 Penguin edition his brother, in the preface, quotes a critic, possibly *H.G. Wells,* who had written the introduction of the 1919 edition, as saying 'it seems that "Barbellion" was a man with a skin too few'. After reading the book it seems likely that *Barbellion* was trying to convey a message to posterity. His 'disappointment' would certainly be much less if the fine nuances of his writing were read today by physicians, neurologists, general practitioners and nurses and thereby enabling them to help their patients by understanding them better.

The third pioneer was *Inman* [1948] who, a few years before he died at a great age, told the author how he had developed retrobulbar neuritis when aged about 40 within a short time of his brother's death from MS. He recognised its prognostic significance as well as its relationship to the death of the brother. This led him to cross Europe to Hungary to consult *Ferenczi,* one of the early psychoanalysts. Subsequently, *Inman* combined opthalmology with the practice of psychoanalysis, and died over 50 years later without recognisable recurrence of retrobulbar neuritis or other manifestation of MS. His surviving relatives have given their permission for this important piece of medical history to be recorded for the first time. On this basis *Ferenczi* may have been the first person to treat MS by psychotherapy, but *Inman's* 1948 article, describing the case of Miss X whom he saw in 1931, shows that he himself was not far behind. Reports by *Langworthy* et al. [1941], *Grinker* et al. [1950], *Harrower* [1950], *Jonez* [1951], *Paulley* [1952], *Philippopoulos* et al. [1958], *Groen* et al. [1967], *Mei-Tal* et al. [1970], and *Paulley* [1976, 1977] all pointed to a definitive emotional vulnerability in MS patients as outlined in this chapter, and summed up by *Philippopoulos* as 'emotional and psychosexual immaturity due to early frustrations and deprivations leading to an infantilisation of character formation ...'. Most of the above reports also make reference to a time relationship to life events epitomising separation and/or engulfment so close 'that the connection ... can hardly be doubted' [*Philippopoulos* et al., 1958]. However, while the potential for psychological management or psychotherapy was almost certainly perceived by these observers few appear to have attempted it. *Inman* certainly did with Miss X and advised full psychoanalysis, but it was *Langworthy* [1947] who first described the essentials of psychotherapy for these patients. 'The hope of therapy is to influence recently acquired abnormalities and prevent the development of further symptoms. These patients show a great need for a physician to interest himself in their problem. They tend to relate themselves to him in the same passive and childish emotional pattern which they have shown to other significant people in their lives. The physicians's problem is to challenge this attitude ... and endeavour to help the patient towards a more mature and satisfactory relationship.' *Jonez* [1951] in a large series also advocated psychotherapy and *Aring* [1965] certainly predicted psychological management. *Groen* et al. [1967] said that 'treatment is best maintained in the form of continuous relationship with the therapist; in a few cases we have seen during such treatment remarkable remissions.' The author described his own approach to psychological management in MS in 1976 and 1977. Since then there have been 2 case reports detailing psychotherapeutic intervention by *Hunyadi-Buzas* [1981] and *Caliezi* [1981], both complement what has been said, and also raise important points of detail in management. The evidence reviewed in this chapter emphasises that while the pathogenesis of MS remains elusive, consideration of emotional stress is of importance and seems relevant to our understanding and management of this neurological disease.

References

Arnason, B.G.W.: 'Multiple sclerosis' research, p. 238. M.R.C. Symp. (HMSO London 1975).

Aring, C.D.: Observations on multiple sclerosis and conversion hysteria. Brain. 88: 663–674 (1965).

Barbellion, W.N.R. (Pseudonym): Cummings, B.F.: The journal of a disappointed man (Chatto & Windus, London 1919/Penguin Books, Harmondsworth 1948).

Brown, G.W.: Methodological research on stressful life events; in Dohrenwend, Dohrenwend, Stressful life events (Wiley, New York 1974).

Bulandra, R.; Siferescu, S.: Considerations of psychical disturbances in mutliple sclerosis. Neurol. Psychiat. Neurochir. 13: 547–551 (1968).

Caliezi, J.M.: Multiple sclerosis – a depressive syndrome? Report on the course of psychotherapy. Psychosom. Med. Psychoanal. 27: 168–179 (1981).

Caplan, L.R.; Nadelson, T.: Multiple sclerosis and hysteria. J. Am. med. Ass. 243: 2418–2421 (1980).

Charcot, J.M.: Lectures on the diseases of the nervous system, pp. 194–195 (New Sydenham Society, 1877).

Cottrell, S.S.; Wilson, S.A.K.: The affective symptomatology of disseminated sclerosis. A study of 100 cases. J. Neurol. Psychopathol. 7: 1–30 (1926).

Cummings, B.F.: See Barbellion, 1948.

Davison, K.; Bagley, C.R.: Schizophrenia-like psychoses associated with organic disorders of the central nervous system; in Heatherington, Current problems in neuropsychiatry (Headley Bros., Kent 1969).

Engel, G.L.: Studies of ulcerative colitis. Am. J. dig. Dis. 3: 315 (1958).

Erikson, E. Identity with the life cycle. Psychol. Issues Monogr. 1: (1959).

Este, A.F. d': Manuscript bok RCP London; cited by Firth, First account of multiple sclerosis. Proc. R. Soc. Med. 34: 381–384 (1941).

Freud, S.: The ego and the id. Collected works (Institute of Psychoanalysis and Hogarth Press, London 1923–1925).

Freud, S.: Formulations regarding the two principles in mental functions. Collected papers, part 1V (Institute of Psychoanalysis and Hogarth Press, London 1922).

Goldberg, D.A.: A psychiatric study of patients with diseases of the small intestine. Gut 11: 459–465 (1970).

Grinker, R.G.; Ham, G.C.; Robbins, F.: Some psychodynamic factors in multiple sclerosis. A. Res. Publ. nerv. ment. Dis. *28:* 456–459 (1950).
Groen, J.J.; Prick, J.J.G.; Bastiaans, J.: Psychosomatic aspects of multiple sclerosis. V11 Eur. Conf. Psychosomatic Res. Acta Med. Psychosom. *1967:* 3–6.
Harrower, M.R.: The results of psychometric and personality tests in multiple sclerosis. A. Res. Publ. nerv. ment. dis. *28:* 461 (1950).
Hollender, A.U.; Steckler, P.P.: Multiple sclerosis and schizophrenia. Psychiat. Med. *3:* 251–257 (1972).
Hunyadi-Buzas, E.: A psychosomatic attitude toward multiple sclerosis. Praxis *70:* 866–868 (1981).
Inman, W.S.: Can emotional conflict induce disseminated sclerosis? Br. J. med. Psychol. *12:* 135–154 (1948).
Jonez, H.D.: Psychotherapy in mutliple sclerosis. Ann. Allergy *9:* 653–659 (1951).
Kemp, K.; Lion, J.R.; Magnam, G.: Lithium in treatment of manic patient with multiple sclerosis. Dis. nerv. Syst. *3:* 210–211 (1977).
Klein, M.: The psychoanalysis of children (Hogarth Press and Institute of Psychoanalysis, London 1932).
Langworthy, O.R.: Relation of personality problems to onset and progress of multiple sclerosis. Archs Neurol. Psychiat., Chicago *59:* 13–28 (1947).
Lemere, F.: Psychiatric disorders in mutliple sclerosis. Am. J. Psychiat., suppl., pp. 55–58 (1966).
Mapelli, C.; Ramelli, E.: Manic symptoms with multiple sclerosis: secondary mania. Acta psychiat. belg. *81:* 337–339 (1981)
Marty, P.; de M'Uzan: La pensée operatoire. Rev. fr. Psychoanal *27;* suppl., p. 1345 (1963).
Matthews, W.B.: Multiple sclerosis presenting with acute remitting psychiatric symptoms. J Neurol. Neurosurg. Psychiat. *42:* 859–863 (1979).
Mei-Tal, V.; Meyerowitz, S.; Engel, G.L.: The role of psychological process in a somatic disorder: mutliple sclerosis. Psychosom. Med. *32:* 67–86 (1969).
Monaco, F.; Mutani, R.; Piredda, S.; Senini, A.: Psychotic onset of multiple sclerosis. Ital. J. neurol. sci. *4:* 279–280 (1980).
Moron, R.; Bonnefous, L.: Mania and multiple sclerosis. Annls méd. psychol. *1:* 119–128 (1976).
Nemiah, J.C.: Psychology and psychosomatic illness. Reflections on theory and research methodology. Psychother. Psychothom. *22:* 106–111 (1973).
Osuch, Z.: Pseudoneurasthenic syndrome as an initial state of multiple sclerosis. Wiad.-Lek. *27:* 21–24 (1974).
Paulley, J.W.: Multiple sclerosis. Lancet *i:* 1305 (1952).
Paulley, J.W.: The psychological management of multiple sclerosis. An overview. Psychother. Psychosom. *27:* 26–40 (1976–77).
Paulley, J.W.: The psychological management of multiple sclerosis. Practitioner *218:* 100–195 (1977).
Paulley, J.W.: Prise en charge psychologique des malades atteints de colite ulcereuse. Méd. Hyg. *39:* 269–273 (1981).
Paulley, J.W.: Pathological mourning. A key factor in the psychopathogenesis of autoimmune disorders. Psychother. Psychosom. *40:* 181–190 (1983).
Payk, T.R.: Psychological particulars in patients with multiple sclerosis. Nervenarzt *44:* 378–380 (1973).

Peselow, E.D.; Deutsch, S.I.; Fieve, R.R.; Kaufman, M.: Coexistent manic symptoms and multiple sclerosis. Psychosomatics 22: 824–825 (1981).

Philippopoulos, G.G.; Witower, E.D.; Cousinean, A.: The etiologic significance of emotional factors in onset and exacerbations of multiple sclerosis. Psychosom. Med. 20: 458–474 (1958).

Pratt, R.T.C.: An investigation of the psychiatric aspects of disseminated sclerosis. J. Neurol. Neurosurg. Psychiat. 14: 326–336 (1951).

Putman, J.T.: Studies in multiple sclerosis. VIII. Etiologic factors in multiple sclerosis. Ann. intern. Med. 9: 854–863 (1936).

Ruesch, J.: The infantile personality: the core problem of psychosomatic medicine. Psychosom. Med. 10: 134–144 (1948).

Runge, W.: Bumke's Handbuch der Geisteskrankheiten. 7: 616 (1928).

Sai-Halasz, A.: Psychic alterations in obsessional sclerosis. Mschr. Psychiat. Neurol. 132: 129–154 (1956).

Salguero, L.F.; Itabashi, H.H.; Gutierrez, N.B.: Childhood multiple sclerosis psychotic manifestations. J. Neurosurg. Psychiat. 32: 572–579 (1969).

Sifneos, P.E.: The prevalence of 'alexithymic' characteristics in psychosomatic patients. Psychother. Psychosom. 22: 255–262 (1973).

Smith, G.: Fear versus paralysis. Cited by Paylley, 1976 (Observer, London, January 12, 1975).

Surridge, D.: An investigation into some psychiatric aspects of multiple sclerosis. Br. J. Psychiat. 155: 749–764 (1969).

Trimble, M.R.; Grant, I.: Psychiatric aspects of multiple sclerosis; in Benson, Psychiatric aspects of neurologic disease, vol. 2 (Gruner & Stratton, New York 1983).

Warren, S.; Green, S.; Warren, K.G.: Emotional stress and the development of multiple sclerosis: case-control evidence of a relationship. J. chron. Dis. 35: 821–831 (1982).

Wender, M.; Dominik, W.: Psychological examination in patients with multiple sclerosis. Psychiat. Neurol. Med. Psychol. 24: 364–392 (1972).

Whitlock, F.A.; Siskind, M.A.: Depression as a major symptom of multiple sclerosis. J. Neurol. neurosurg. Psychiat. 43: 861–865 (1980).

Dr. J.W. Paulley, 51 Anglesey Road, Ipswich IPI 3PJ (UK).

6. Psychosomatic Aspects of Movement Disorders

J.L. Cummings[1]

Neurobehavior Unit, West Los Angeles VAMC (Brentwood Division) and
Department of Neurology UCLA School of Medicine, Los Angeles, Calif., USA

Disturbances of motility are common accompaniments of psychiatric disorders such as schizophrenia, mania, depression, anxiety, and obsessive-compulsive disorders. On the other hand, extrapyramidal diseases (Parkinson's disease, Huntington's disease, etc.) are commonly associated with a rich and diverse spectrum of neuropsychiatric alterations including dementia, affective disorders, schizophrenia-like illnesses, and obsessive-compulsive behavior. This reciprocal relationship suggests that behavioral and motor phenomena may share common pathophysiologic mechanisms, but this correlation has recieved relatively little systematic study. Thus, the bradykinesia, rigidity and tremor of Parkinsonian syndromes, the hyperkinesia of the choreic disorders, and the tics of Gilles de la Tourette syndrome have been emphasized as the main elements of these extrapyramidal disorders, whereas the mental status alterations that commonly accompany them have been minimized. Likewise, investigations of schizophrenia have emphasized delusions, hallucinations, and formal thought disorder and have paid less attention to the gestures, mannerisms, stereotypies, and bizarre alterations of gait and posture that may be manifest in some schizophrenic patients. The impact of psychological and environmental events on the motor manifestations of various diseases has likewise received scant attention. Tremors and tics may be markedly worsened by anxiety; tics and tardive dyskinesia are much more evident during the depressed than during euthymic or manic periods of manic depressive illnesses; and tics and dyskinesias may be volitionally controlled for short periods of time. These observations demonstrate the important influence

---

[1] This project was supported by the Veterans Administration. *Johanne Sandilands* and *Norene Hiekel* prepared the manuscript.

Table I. Psychiatric disturbances associated with extrapyramidal diseases

Extrapyramidal disease	Associated psychiatric disorder
Postencephalitic Parkinson's disease	schizophrenia-like illness
	mania
	depression
	conduct disorder
	obsessive-compulsive disorder
Idiopathic Parkinson's disease	depression
Huntington's disease	depression
	mania
	schizophrenia-like illness
Wilson's disease	depression
	mania
	schizophrenia-like illness
Idiopathic basal ganglia calcification	schizophrenia-like illness
Gilles de la Tourette syndrome	obsessive-compulsive disorder
Spinocerebellar degeneration	schizophrenia-like psychosis
	depression
Progressive supranuclear palsy	depression
Meige's syndrome	depression
	obsessive-compulsive disorder
Tardive dyskinesia	psychosis?

of psychological and environmental circumstances on motor function and reveal the unique bond between the psychological state of the individual and his motor performance.

Recent anatomical and neurochemical discoveries provide a framework for understanding the link between psychological and motor activity. Sizeable connections between the cerebral cortical mantle and the basal ganglia have been delineated and important tracts connecting the limbic system with the basal ganglia have also been described. These projections unite the cortical, limbic, and subcortical structures into a cohesive system mediating motivation, mood, and motion. Likewise, dopaminergic and noradrenergic transmitters, thought to be disturbed in the psychoses and affective disorders, have been found to originate in, traverse through, and take part in the function of the subcortical structures. Thus, the identical neurotransmitters implicated in the major psychiatric illnesses are also affected in the extrapyramidal disorders.

These observations challenge the view of extrapyramidal diseases as 'movement disorders' and of psychiatric illnesses as 'functional' disturbances and suggest that they be seen as disorders of psychomotility with central nervous system dysfunction expressed in both the motoric and psychological realms. This chapter will discuss 10 extrapyramidal disorders – postencephalitic Parkinson's disease, idiopathic Parkinson's disease, Huntington's disease, Wilson's disease, idiopathic calcification of the basal ganglia, Gilles de la Tourette syndrome, spinocerebellar degenerations, progressive supranuclear palsy, Meige's syndrome, and tardive dyskinesia (table I) – from this perspective. Psychosomatic aspects of each syndrome will be emphasized. Five idiopathic psychiatric disorders – schizophrenia, mania, depression, anxiety, and obsessive-compulsive disorder – will also be presented and their motoric manifestations described. The subcortical anatomical and neurochemical systems implicated in both extrapyramidal and behavioral disturbances will also be discussed. To present a comprehensive view, 'psychosomatic' will be broadly interpreted to include both the consequences of dysfunction of subcortical structures for psychological activity and the influence of psychological and environmental activity on the functions of the motor system.

Extrapyramidal Disorders

Parkinson's Disease

Postencephalitic Parkinson's disease (PEPD), though rare today, remains a classic example of a subcortical disease with major ramifications in both motor and psychological spheres. PEPD resulted from an acute viral encephalitis (von Economo's encephalitis, encephalitis lethargica) that occurred in epidemic proportions between 1919 and 1926. The acute encephalitic illness was characterized by somnolence, ocular motor and limb paralyses, extrapyramidal disturbances, sensory changes, and autonomic dysfunction [*Barker,* 1921; *Riley,* 1930]. These symptoms were accompanied by a variety of neuropsychiatric alterations including hyperkinetic disorders, euphoria, schizophrenia-like psychoses, delirium, depression, emotional instability, and irritability [*Hohman,* 1921; *Sandy,* 1920]. Survivors of encephalitis either entered directly into a postencephalitic Parkinsonian state or enjoyed an interval recovery period lasting months to years before a Parkinsonian syndrome supervened. 80% of those surviving the encephalitis developed PEPD within 10 years [*Duvoisin and Yahr,* 1965].

Like the acute encephalitis, PEPD was associated with a diverse array of psychiatric disturbances including schizophrenia-like illnesses, mania, conduct disorders, depression, and obsessive-compulsive disorders (table I) [*Bromberg*, 1930; *Fairweather*, 1947; *Jelliffe*, 1929; *Meninger*, 1926]. Striking as it did simultaneously with the delivery of *Freud's* [1920] introductory psychoanalytic lectures in Vienna, encephalitis lethargica and its postencephalitic psychomotility disorders played an essential role in focusing attention on the relationship between brain disturbances and psychiatric abnormalities at a time when psychodynamic explanations of behavior were gaining increasing popularity.

The pathology of PEPD consisted of a chronic inflammatory infiltration with glial proliferation and cell loss in the rostral brainstem, hypothalamus, subthalamus, globus pallidus, and to a lesser extent the neostriatum [*Buzzard and Greenfield*, 1919; *Eaves and Crall*, 1930–1931; *McAlpine*, 1923].

Idiopathic Parkinson's disease (IPD) or paralysis agitans, does not produce the dramatic psychiatric alterations associated with PEPD, but depression is prominent among its clinical manifestations. Depression may be the presenting feature of IPD, and clinically significant depression occurs in 40–60% of IPD patients [*Brown and Wilson*, 1972; *Celesia and Wanamaker*, 1972; *Jackson* et al., 1923; *Mindham*, 1970]. The incidence of depression in IPD has been compared with that occurring in other patients with comparable degrees of motoric disability – paraplegics, medically ill patients, patients with mixed neurological and orthopedic disorders – and found to be significantly greater among those with IPD [*Horn*, 1974; *Robins*, 1976; *Warburton*, 1967]. This indicates that the depression cannot be completely accounted for on the basis of a reaction to the physical handicap and suggests that it is an integral component of the IPD syndrome. Tricyclic antidepressants usually relieve the depression associated with IPD and have little effect on the movement disorder, whereas levodopa facilitates motor activity and is a poor antidepressant [*Andersen*, 1980; *Laitinen*, 1969; *Mindham* et al., 1976; *Strang*, 1965]. Electroconvulsive therapy has a salutary effect on both expressions of IPD, but the improvement in mood is more lasting [*Asnis*, 1977; *Lebensohn and Jenkins*, 1975].

The expression of the movement disorder of IPD is also intimately linked to the emotional state of the individual. Tremor is increased by emotional stress, and the mobility of the patient may be profoundly affected by environmental circumstances [*Marsden and Owen*, 1967]. The 'central paradox' of IPD is the ability of some patients, rigid and akinetic for years, to suddenly run for safety when an emergency arises, only to relapse into a motionless state when the emergency is passed [*Schwab and Zieper,* 1965; *Yakovlev,* 1966]. Such observations demonstrate the constant interplay between the emotional and motor realms in IPD.

Pathologically, IPD exhibits striking loss of neurons in the substantia nigra, locus coeruleus and other pigmented brain stem nuclei, and the hypothalamus. Remaining neurons contain an excessive number of Lewy bodies [*Den Hartog Jager and Bethlem,* 1960; *Greenfield and Bosanquet, 1953; Langston and Forno,* 1978]. In addition to involvement of the nigrostriatal dopamine pathway through degeneration of nigral neurons, there is also loss of dopaminergic projections to limbic system cortex from the midbrain ventral tegmental area [*Javoy-Agid and Agid,* 1980; *Price* et al., 1978]. Thus, the pathology of IPD involves not only the nigrostriatal pathways classically thought to mediate the movement disturbance, but also involves hypothalamus and limbic cortex concerned with the mediation of motivation and mood.

Huntington's Disease

In his original description of 'hereditary chorea' in 1872, *George Huntington* commented on the propensity of afflicted individuals to commit suicide. This observation has been amply confirmed and an increased prevalence of clinically significant affective disorders among Huntington's disease (HD) patients is now well recognized. *Dewhurst* et al. [1969], in a study of 80 HD patients, found that affective disorders were present in a majority of patients and were the principal reason for hospital admission in approximately 20%. The affective disorder may be depression or may be a bipolar disorder with cyclical mood elevation and depression [*Dewhurst* et al., 1969; *Folstein* et al., 1979; *McHugh and Folstein,* 1975]. The occurrence of both mania and depression in patients with HD implies that the affective alterations are not reactive but are a neurobiologic expression of the subcortical disease process. The depression associated with HD frequently responds to conventional therapy with tricyclic antidepressants [*Whittier* et al., 1961; *Shoulson,* 1981].

In addition to affective disturbances, a schizophrenia-like illness with hallucinations and delusions, has also been observed in HD patients [*Caine and Shoulson,* 1983; *Garron,* 1973; *McHugh and Folstein,* 1975; *Rosenbaum,* 1941]. The schizophrenia-like illness and the affective disorders are most common in the early stages of HD and recede as the dementia advances.

As in Parkinson's disease, the motor manifestations of HD worsen with anxiety, and some cases have become apparent only when stressful circumstances exaggerated the choreiform movements [*Korenyi* et al., 1972].

Pathologically, there is pronounced cell loss in the caudate nucleus and putamen of HD patients and less conspicuous involvement of the thalamus, globus pallidus, claustrum, and subthalamic nuclei. Pathological changes in the cortex of the frontal lobe are variable [*Corsellis*, 1976; *Cummings and Benson*, 1983].

Wilson's Disease

Wilson's disease manifests a spectrum of psychopathology similar to that observed in HD. Depression and mania have been reported in Wilson's disease patients [*Pandy* et al., 1981; *Scheinberg and Sternlieb*, 1984], and a schizophrenia-like psychosis with hallucinations and delusions is not uncommon [*Beard*, 1959; *Gysin and Cooke*, 1950; *Jackson and Immerman*, 1919; *Scheinberg and Steinlieb*, 1984].

At autopsy, there are pronounced abnormalities (cell loss, gliosis) in the putamen and less severe changes in the globus pallidus, subthalamic nuclei, caudate nuclei, dentate nuclei, frontal lobe cortex, and cerebral and cerebellar white matter [*Cummings and Benson*, 1983; *Scheinberg and Sternlieb*, 1984].

Idiopathic Basal Ganglia Calcification

Idiopathic basal ganglia calcification (IBGC) is a rare disorder that may present in one of two ways: (1) as a schizophrenia-like psychosis, or (2) as a progressive dementing illness with Parkinsonism or choreoathetosis [*Cummings* et al., 1983]. The schizophrenia-like disorder is manifested by hallucinations, delusions, and thought disorder [*Bruyn* et al., 1964; *Cummings* et al., 1983; *Francis*, 1979; *Kalamboukis and Molling*, 1962; *Kasanin and Crank*, 1935]. The average age at onset of the psychosis is 30 years compared with 50 years for the dementia and extrapyramidal disturbance. Those with psychosis eventually develop the intellectual impairment and movement disorder noted in the late-onset variety.

Pathological alterations in IBGC include excessive calcium deposition, cell loss and gliosis in the globus pallidus, putamen, thalamus, corona radiata, dentate nuclei, and cerebral and cerebellar white matter. The calcification is concentrated in the walls of arteries and capillaries and in the perivascular parenchyma of both gray and white matter [*Adachi* et al.,

1968; *Friede* et al., 1961; *Kasanin and Crank,* 1935; *Kalamboukis and Molling* 1962; *Neumann,* 1963].

Gilles de la Tourette Syndrome

Gilles de la Tourette syndrome (GTS) is an idiopathic chronic multiple tic syndrome that has its onset between ages 2 and 15 years, is manifested by multiple somatic tics and involuntary vocalizations, and has a life-long waxing and waning course [*Shapiro* et al., 1978]. Additional symptoms that may occur but are not essential to the diagnosis include coprolalia, copropraxia, echolalia, echopraxia, and palilalia.

Obsessions and compulsions have been noted to occur with increased frequency among GTS patients since Tourette first described the syndrome. Estimates of the prevalence of obsessive-compulsive disorder in GTS have varied between 12 and 90% depending on the sample studied and the ascertainment methods [*Corbett* et al., 1969; *Fernando,* 1967; *Nee* et al., 1980, 1982; *Montgomery* et al., 1982; *Morphew and Sim,* 1969]. Using a structured questionnaire, we found that 54% of GTS patients endorsed as many items as patients with idiopathic obsessive-compulsive disorder. Thus, obsessions and compulsions appear to be a frequent manifestation of CNS dysfunction in GTS and may represent the severe end of a spectrum of symptoms stretching from simple tics through complex tics to disabling compulsions and ritualistic behavior.

In addition to the apparent association of obsessions and compulsions with the neurological dysfunction, the symptoms of GTS are also subject to a variety of environmental, emotional, and volitonal influences. In most cases, tics can be voluntarily controlled for short periods of time [*Shapiro* et al., 1978]. Patients may suppress the tics for up to an hour or more, but a subjective sense of tension mounts during the controlled period and is relieved only by allowing the tics to reassert themselves. This degree of volitional control indicates that the disordered neuronal function of GTS is not completely autonomous but is subject to temporary control by intact portions of the nervous system. In addition to volitional control, other factors that influence the symptoms of GTS include stress and depression. Stressful situations and anxiety increase the frequency of tics. Tics are also more frequent during depressed than during euthymic periods [*Sweeney* et al., 1978].

The few autopsy studies of GTS patients have been unrevealing, but a variety of pharmacological, biochemical, and clinical observations suggest that the underlying abnormality is a hyperactivity of striatal and/or limbic dopamine systems [*Singer*, 1982]. Dopaminergic dysfunction is suggested by the success of dopamine-blocking agents in controlling the symptoms of GTS, by the aggravation of GTS by monoaminergic stimulants, and by the identification of abnormal monoaminergic metabolites in the cerebrospinal fluid of GTS patients [*Butler* et al., 1979; *Cohen* et al., 1978; *Golden*, 1977; *Messifia* et al., 1971; *Shapiro* et al., 1978, *Singer* et al., 1982]. The origin of tics from subcortical dysfunction is also supported by neurophysiological studies demonstrating that they are not preceded by cortically-mediated premovement potentials that preface normal volitional motor activity [*Obeso* et al., 1981]. Finally, the occurrence of extrapyramidal features in GTS (dystonia, choreoathetosis, oculogyric-like movements), and the existence of GTS symptoms in known basal ganglia disorders (postencephalitic Parkinsonism, carbon monoxide encephalopathy, tardive dyskinesia) also suggest that GTS is a product of dysfunction of subcortical structures [*Frankel and Cummings*, 1984; *Klawans* et al., 1978; *Pulst* et al., 1983; *Wohlfart* et al., 1961]. Thus, the tics and vocalizations as well as the obsessions and compulsions appear to result from unrestrained hyperfunction of subcortical systems.

Spinocerebellar Degenerations

Spinocerebellar degenerations are a diverse group of degenerative central nervous system disorders variably involving the spinal cord, brain stem, and cerebellum, and occasionally extending to affect the thalamus, subthalamic structures and basal ganglia. The neuropsychiatric disorders correlated with these conditions have not been systematically studied, but accumulated reports of individual cases and affected families suggest an association with depression and a schizophrenia-like psychosis [*Chandler and Begin*, 1956; *Davies*, 1949; *Richards* et al., 1974, *Shepherd*, 1955].

Progressive Supranuclear Palsy

Progressive supranuclear palsy (PSP) is a progressive degenerative disorder characterized by axial rigidity, pseudobulbar palsy, supranuclear gaze palsy, and dementia [*Steele*, 1972; *Steele* et al., 1964]. In addition to deterioration of intellectual function, PSP patients are also commonly depressed [*Albert* et al., 1974; *Jackson* et al., 1983; *Janati and Appel*, 1984], and the depression may respond to treatment with tricyclic antidepressants [*Kvale*, 1982].

Pathological studies in PSP reveal cell loss, gliosis, neurofibrillary tangles, granulovacuolar degeneration, and demyelination involving the basal ganglia, parts of the thalamus, the brain stem, and the cerebellum. The most severely affected structures include the globus pallidus, subthalamic nucleus, red nucleus, substantia nigra, superior colliculi, periaqueductal gray matter, pontine tegmentum, and the dentate nucleus [*Steele,* 1972; *Steele* et al., 1964].

Meige's Syndrome

Meige's Syndrome is an idiopathic extrapyramidal disorder manifested by blepharospasm, oromandibular dystonia, or both. In some cases there are associated dystonic movements of the neck, upper limbs, or respiratory muscles [*Marsden,* 1976; *Tolosa,* 1981; *Tolosa and Klawans,* 1979]. Psychiatric disturbances noted in association with Meige's Syndrome include depression and obsessive-compulsive symptoms [*Ashizawa* et al., 1980; *Jankovic and Ford,* 1983; *Tolosa,* 1981].

Autopsy findings in Meige's syndrome have been variable, with some investigators unable to find any alterations and others identifying cell loss and gliosis in the caudate and putamen [*Altrocchi and Forno,* 1983; *Garcia-Albea* et al., 1981]. Pharmacologic evidence suggests that the syndrome results from an imbalance of subcortical cholinergic and dopaminergic functions [*Casey,* 1980; *Tolosa and Lai,* 1979].

Tardive Dyskinesia

Tardive dyskinesia (TD) is an extrapyramidal syndrome manifested primarily by orofacial-lingual dyskinesia with variable involvement of limbs and truncal musculature. It is a product of long-term treatment with neuroleptic agents and develops in 15–25% of patients chronically exposed to these agents [*Jeste and Wyatt,* 1982]. Like GTS and Meige's syndrome, no consistent neuropathology has been found in TD but pharmacological studies suggest that the chronic dopamine receptor blockade by neuroleptic agents induces a compensatory receptor hypersensitivity and consequent extrapyramidal hyperactivity [*Gerlach* et al., 1974; *Tarsy and Baldessarini,* 1977].

Although a psychiatric counterpart of tardive dyskinesia is not yet widely accepted, several investigators have suggested that there is a tardive psychosis that results from dopamine receptor hypersensitivity in the mesolimbic dopamine system [*Chouinard and Jones,* 1980; *Davis and Rosenberg,* 1979]. Other psychosomatic aspects of TD, however, are less controversial. Like GTS, TD is exaccerbated by stress and by depression and can be volitionally suppressed on a temporary basis [*Cutler* et al., 1981; *Weiner and Werner,* 1982].

Movement Disorders in Psychiatric Illnesses

Schizophrenia

Movement abnormalities are not uncommon in schizophrenia and may include mannerisms, stereotypies, a variety of catatonic behaviors, and bizarre alterations of posture and gait [*Hamilton,* 1984; *Marsden* et al., 1975]. Mannerisms are excerpts of purposeful behavior performed in an unusual way, whereas stereotypies are purposeless behaviors repeated in an unvarying pattern. These movements may involve the fingers, arms, legs, trunk, or face and may be difficult to distinguish from tardive dyskinesia though they were described before the introduction of neuroleptic agents and may be observed prior to the administration of these drugs [*Cunningham and Johnstone,* 1982]. Movement abnormalities in schizophrenia are associated with a poor prognosis for the disorder [*Yarden and Discipio,* 1971].

The neuropathological basis of schizophrenia has not been determined, but psychopharmacological evidence suggests that the disorder is mediated by dopaminergic neurotransmitter systems, and the few available neuropathologic studies have found abnormalities in dopamine-rich limbic and subcortical sites [*Stevens,* 1982].

Affective Disorders

Like schizophrenia, mania has both cognitive and motoric manifestations. The patients became physically hyperactive, pacing or running about and getting involved in numerous activities. Their speech is rapid and their affective expression exaggerated [*Marsden* et al., 1975]. Depression, on the other hand, is characterized by psychomotor retardation, bowed posture, shuffling gait, sparse verbal output, and hypophonia [*Cummings and Benson,* 1983; *Marsden* et al., 1975]. Catatonic behavior can occur in both mania and depression [*Taylor and Abrams,* 1977].

The success of tricyclic antidepressants and monoamine oxidase inhibitors in the treatment of depression and the occasional induction of a manic episode by these agents suggests a major role for noradrenergic mechanisms in the pathogenesis of affective disorders with contributions from serotonergic and, perhaps, dopaminergic systems in some cases [*Schildkraut,* 1970].

Anxiety

The most apparent motor manifestation of anxiety is tremor. The tremor is typically a high frequency low amplitude action tremor that disappears or is minimal at rest and is exaggerated by purposeful activities. Other common motor alterations in anxiety include pacing, widening of the palpebral fissures, raising the eyebrows and furrowing the forehead, and tachypnea [*Left and Isaacs,* 1981].

The pathophysiology of anxiety has received less study than the mechanisms underlying psychosis, but the production of anxiety by amphetamines and sympathomimetic agents and the reversal of many of the symptoms by adrenergic blocking agents again suggests that noradrenergic hyperactivity is responsible for many of the physiologic aspects of anxiety. Gamma-aminobutyric acid (Gaba) and serotonin have also been implicated in the pathogenesis of anxiety [*Hoehn-Saric,* 1982], and links between monoamines, Gaba, and the limbic forebrain in experimental anxiety are discussed by *Gray* in chapter 1.

Obsessive-Compulsive Disorder

Obsessive-compulsive disorder is a rare idiopathic psychiatric disorder characterized by recurrent ego-dystonic ideas, thoughts, images, or impulses (obsessions) and/or stereotyped, irresistable, repetitive behaviors (compulsions) [Diagnostic and Statistical Manual, 1980]. The compulsions include forced touching, avoidance manoeuvers, and ritualistic behaviors that impart an unusual and sometimes alien quality to the patient's motor behavior.

The biochemical basis of obsessions and compulsions is unknown, but their prominence in Gilles de la Tourette syndrome, Meige's syndrome and PEPD suggests a relationship to hyperdopaminergic states.

Anatomical Connections of the Basal Ganglia

The anatomical connections of the basal ganglia provide some insight into why extrapyramidal disorders are so frequently accompanied by psychiatric disturbances and why the movement abnormalities of extrapyramidal diseases are subject to alteration by stress, depression, or

Table II. Projections from limbic system structures to components of the extrapyramidal system [Nauta, 1982; Nauta and Domesick, 1978].

Limbic system structure	Extrapyramidal system target
Amygdala	striatum
	nucleus accumbens
Hippocampus	striatum
	nucleus accumbens
Cingulate cortex	striatum
Ventral tegmental area	striatum
Hypothalamus	substantia nigra

temporary volitional control. Particularly important in this regard are the connections between the limbic system and the basal ganglia (table II). A number of limbic projections to the striatum have been mapped, including afferents from the ventral tegmental area of the midbrain, amygdala, hippocampus, and cingulate cortex (fig. 1). Moreover, it has been discovered that only a small portion of the head of the caudate is devoted solely to somato-motor functions, whereas the majority of the striatum receives afferents from both the limbic system and the prefrontal cortex [Nauta, 1982]. In addition to these profuse limbic projections to the striatum, other limbic-subcortical intersections include hippocampal and amygdaloid projections to the nucleus accumbens (a striatal nucleus), and hypothalamic projections via the medial forebrain bundle to the substantia nigra (fig. 1) [Nauta and Domesick, 1978]. Thus, striatal, septal, and nigral nuclei of the extrapyramidal system receive a rich input from the limbic system creating a convergence of systems mediating motivation and motion and providing an anatomical avenue for the influence of the emotional state on motor function.

The other major input to the extrapyramidal system is from the cerebral cortex. Once thought to interact mainly with primary motor cortex, the basal ganglia are now known to receive projections from wide areas of the neocortex. All parts of the cortex send fibers to the striatum in a topographically organized pattern. The largest projections come from frontal and parietal association cortices, and there are robust afferents from motor and somatosensory areas [Kemp and Powell, 1970]. These neocortical projections convey environmentally generated sensory impulses and

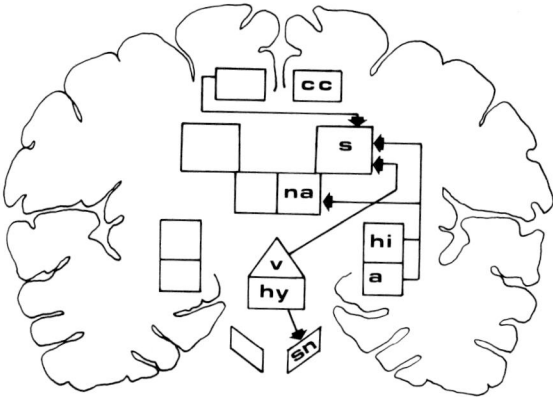

Fig. 1. Schematic representation of the projections from limbic to extrapyramidal structures. A=Amygdala; CC=cingulate cortex; Hi=hippocampus; Hy=hypothalamus; NA=nucleus accumbens; S=striatum; SN=substantia nigra; V=ventral tegmental area.

volitionally generated motor impulses to the striatum and provide an anatomical basis for sensory and volitional influences on the motor manifestations of extrapyramidal diseases.

Subcortical Neurochemical Systems

Four neurotransmitters have been implicated most often in the extrapyramidal syndromes and their associated behavioral disturbances: dopamine, noradrenaline, serotonin, and gamma-aminobutyric acid (Gaba) (table III). Dopaminergic pathways include a nigrostriatal connection, a mesolimbic projection, and a tuberoinfundibular pathway. The latter is implicated primarily in neuroendocrinological function. The nigrostriatal pathway originates from dopamine neurons in the pars compacta of the substantia nigra and projects to striatal receptors. The mesolimbic dopaminergic pathway originates in the ventral tegmental area and projects to the nucleus accumbens, amygdala, limbic portions of the striatum, and areas of the frontal cortex receiving afferents from limbic thalamic nuclei [*Mishra* et al., 1975; *Nauta and Domesick*, 1978; *Ungerstedt*, 1971]. Thus, both limbic and extrapyramidal systems are heavily invested by dopamine projections and involvement of both areas may account for the coincident occurrence of motor and behavioral abnormalities in disorders

Table III. Neurotransmitters involved in the subcortical disorders, their principal origins and destinations, and the disorders in which they have been implicated

Neurotransmitter	Origin	Destination	Associated disease
Dopamine	substantia nigra, ventral tegmental area	striatum, nucleus accumbens, amygdala, limbic striatum, limbic cortex	idiopathic Parkinson's disease, postencephalitic Parkinson's disease, Gilles de la Tourette syndrome, Meige's syndrome, tardive dyskinesia, progressive supranuclear palsy, schizophrenia
Noradrenaline	medulla, pons (locus coeruleus, formatio reticularis)	hypothalamus, nuclei of stria terminalis, septal area, amygdaloid complex, hippocampal formation, cingulate cortex, neocortex	depression, anxiety
Serotonin	midbrain and rostral pontine raphe nuclei	hypothalamus, globus pallidus, septal area, amygdaloid complex, cingulate gyrus	depression
Gaba	interneurons of striatum and substantia nigra		Huntington's disease, anxiety

with disturbed dopamine metabolism such as idiopathic Parkinson's disease, postencephalitic Parkinson's disease, Gilles de la Tourette syndrome, Meige's syndrome, tardive dyskinesia and, possibly, progressive supranuclear palsy. Dopamine is also the primary neurotransmitter implicated in the pathogenesis of schizophrenia.

The principal ascending noradrenergic tracts originate in the medulla and pons (locus coeruleus, formatio reticularis) and project via the medial forebrain bundle to the hypothalamus, limbic forebrain structures (nuclei of stria terminalis, septal area, amygdaloid complex, hippocampal formation, cingulate cortex), and cerebral cortex [Andén et al., 1966; Ungerstedt, 1971]. The highest density of noradrenaline is found in the hypothalamus; the density in the limbic structures is somewhat less; and the lowest concentrations are found in the cerebral cortex [*Snyder,* 1976]. Noradrenaline and dopamine projections share many anatomical features in common including origin in the brain stem and distribution through the medial forebrain bundle to target structures in the cerebral hemispheres. These pathways are vulnerable to disruption by subcortical lesions. Noradrenaline has been implicated as the neurotransmitter most likely to be disturbed in depression [*Schildkraut,* 1970], and involvement of these subcortical noradrenergic pathways may explain the high frequency of mood disorders in subcortical diseases. Noradrenaline, as noted, also plays a role in the pathogenesis of anxiety.

Serotonin has also been implicated in the pathogenesis of depression, and, like dopamine and noradrenaline, it is also manufactured by nuclear groups in the brain stem (midbrain raphe nuclei) and is transported through tracts in the medial forebrain bundle to the hypothalamus, limbic forebrain structures, and cerebral cortex [*Andén* et al., 1966; *Snyder,* 1976; *Ungerstedt,* 1971]. Serotonin pathways share the same anatomical vulnerability to subcortical diseases noted for noradrenaline and dopamine.

Finally, Gaba is preferentially affected in Huntington's disease. Gaba loss presumably accounts for the choreic movements and could play a role in the neuropsychiatric disturbances that frequently accompany HD. Gaba is an inhibitory neurotransmitter of the striatum and substantia nigra [*Lance and McLeod,* 1981].

Conclusions

This review has emphasized that a variety of psychosomatic dimensions are relevent to disturbances of movement. First, diseases of the basal ganglia are frequently accompanied by psychiatric disturbances including schizophrenia-like illnesses, depression, mania and obsessive-compulsive disorders. Second, there is an active commerce between the psychological state of the individual and the motoric expressions of the subcortical diseases. Anxiety, stress, and depression tend to exacerbate movement disorders, whereas relaxation improves them. Some motor disturbances are also subject to considerable voluntary control, at least on a temporary basis. Third, idiopathic psychiatric illnesses such as schizophrenia, affective disorders, anxiety, and obsessive-compulsive disorders commonly have manifestations the motoric realm.

Both anatomical and neurochemical information contributes to understanding the neurobiological bases of the relation between behavioral and motor system abnormalities. Neuroanatomical investigations reveal dense projections from the limbic system to the basal ganglia and suggest that limbic and extrapyramidal structures form a unified system mediating motivation, mood, and motion. Any attempt to dissect the limbic and extrapyramidal functions into separate systems is artificial. Furthermore, the classical anatomical approach of studying gray matter nuclei connected by white matter tracts is being augmented and, in some cases, supplanted by consideration of transmitter systems that connect distant and diverse brain regions into complex unifed organizations. The effects of localized disturbances must be considered not only in terms of local dysfunction but also in terms of distant effects produced by disruption of transmitter transport and distribution. Subcortical diseases are optimally situated anatomically to produce neighborhood effects on basal ganglia and related subcortical structures and also to disrupt transmitter pathways with consequences in distant limbic and striatal structures and neocortex. These same transmitter systems are implicated in the pathogenesis of several of the major psychiatric illnesses, and the combination of anatomical and neurochemical alterations has ramifications for both motor function and behavior. These diseases must be seen as complex disorders of psychomotility in which the underlying neurophysiologic abnormality is manifested in the motor, cognitive, and emotional realms.

References

Adachi, M.; Wellman, K.F.; Volk, B.W.: Histochemical studies on the pathogenesis of idiopathic non-arteriosclerotic cerebral calcification. J. Neuropath. exp. Neurol. *27:* 483–499 (1968).

Albert, M.L.; Feldman, R.G.; Willis, A.L.: The 'subcortical dementia' of progressive supranuclear palsy. J. Neurol. Neurosurg. Psychiat. *37:* 121–130 (1974).

Altrocchi, P.H.; Forno, L.S.: Spontaneous oral-facial dyskinesia: neuropathology of a case. Neurology, Minneap. *33:* 802–805 (1983).

Andén, N.E.; Dahlstrom, A.; Fuxe, K.; Larson, K.; Olson, L.; Ungerstedt, U.: Ascending monoamine neurons to the telencephalon and diencephalon. Acta physiol. scand. *67:* 313–326 (1966).

Anderson, J.; Aabro, E.; Gulmann, N.; Hjelmsted, A.; Pedersen, H.E.: Anti-depressive treatment in Parkinson's disease. Acta neurol. scand. *62:* 210–219 (1980).

Ashizawa, T.; Patten, B.M.; Jankovic, J.: Meige's syndrome. Sth med. J., Nashville *73:* 863–866 (1980).

Asnis, G.: Parkinson's disease, depression, and ECT. A review and case study. Am. J. Psychiat. *134:* 191–194 (1977).

Barker, L.S.: Diagnostic criteria in epidemic encephalitis, and encephalomyelitis. Archs Neurol. Psychiat. *6:* 173–196 (1921).

Beard, A.W.: The association of hepatolenticular degeneration with schizophrenia. Acta psychiat. neurol. *34:* 411–428 (1959).

Bromberg, W.: Mental states in chronic encephalitis. Psychiat. Qt. *4:* 537–566 (1930).

Brown, G.L.; Wilson, W.P.: Parkinsonism and depression. Sth med. J. Nashville *65:* 540–545 (1972).

Bruyn, G.W.; Bots, G.T.A.M.; Staal, A.: Familial bilateral vascular calcification in the central nervous system. Psychiat. Neurol. Neurochir. *67:* 342–376 (1964).

Butler, I.J.; Koslow, S.H.; Seifert, W.E., Jr.; Caprioli, R.M.; Singer H.S.: Biogenic amine metabolism in Tourette syndrome. Ann. Neurol. *6:* 37–39 (1979).

Buzzard, E.F.; Greenfield, J.G.: Lethargic encephalitis: its sequelae and morbid anatomy. Brain *42:* 305–338 (1919).

Caine, E.D.; Shoulson, I.: Psychiatric syndromes in Huntington's disease. Am. J. Psychiat. *140:* 728–733 (1983).

Casey, D.E.: Pharmacology of blepharospasm-oromandibular dystonic syndrome. Neurology, Minneap. *30:* 690–695 (1980).

Celesia, G.G.; Wanamaker, W.M.: Psychiatric disturbances in Parkinson's disease. Dis. nerv. Syst. *33:* 577–583 (1972).

Chandler, J.H.; Bebin, J.: Hereditary cerebellar ataxia. Olivopontocerebellar type. Neurology, Minneap. *6:* 187–195 (1956).

Chouinard, G.; Jones, B.D.: Neuroleptic induced supersensitivity psychosis: clinical and pharmacologic characteristics. Am. J. Psychiat. *137:* 16–21 (1980).

Cohen, D.J.; Shaywitz, B.A.; Caparulo, B.; Young, J.G.; Bowers, M.B., Jr.: Chronic multiple tics of Gilles de la Tourette's disease. Archs gen. Psychiat. *35:* 245–250 (1978).

Corbett, J.A.; Mathews, A.M.; Connell, P.H.; Shapiro, D.A.: Tics and Gilles de la Tourette syndrome. A follow-up study and critical review. Br. J. Psychiat. *115:* 1229–1241 (1969).

Corsellis, J.A.N.: Ageing and the dementias; in Greenfield's neuropathology, pp. 796–848 (Year Book Medical Publishers, Chicago 1976).

Cumming, J.L.; Benson, D.F.: Dementia. A clinical approach (Butterworths, Boston 1983).

Cummings, J.L.; Gosenfeld, L.F.; Houlihan, J.P.; McCaffrey, T.: Neuropsychiatric disturbances associated with idiopathic calcification of the basal ganglia. Biol. Psychiat. *18:* 591–601 (1983).

Cunningham, D.G.; Johnstone, E.C.: Spontaneous involuntary disorders of movement. Archs gen. Psychiat. *39:* 452–461 (1982).

Cutler, N.R.; Post, R.M.; Rey, A.C.; Bunney, W.E., Jr.: Depression-dependent dyskinesias in two cases of manic-depressive illness. New Engl. J. Med. *304:* 1088–1089 (1981).

Davies, D.L.: Psychiatric changes associated with Friedreich's ataxia. J. Neurol. Neurosurg. Psychiat. *12:* 246–250 (1949).

Den Hartog Jager, W.A.; Bethlem, J.: The distribution of Lewy bodies in the central and autonomic nervous systems in idiopathic paralysis agitans. J. Neurol. Neurosurg. Psychiat. *23:* 283–290 (1960).

Dewhurst, K.; Oliver, J.; Trick, K.L.K.; McKnight, A.L.: Neuropsychiatric aspects of Huntington's disease. Confinia neurol. *31:* 258–268 (1969).
Diagnostic and Statistical Manual of Mental Disorders; 3rd ed. (American Psychiatric Association, Washington 1980).
Duvoisin, R.C.; Yahr, M.D.: Encephalitis and Parkinsonism. Archs Neurol. *12:* 227–239 (1965).
Eaves, E.C.; Crall, M.M.: The pituitary and hypothalamic region in chronic epidemic encephalitis. Brain *53:* 56–75 (1930–1931).
Fairweather, D.S.: Psychiatric aspects of the post-encephalitic syndrome. J. ment. Sci. *93:* 201–254 (1947).
Fernando, S.J.M.: Gilles de la Tourette's syndrome. Br. J. Psychiat. *113:* 607–617 (1967).
Folstein, S.E.; Folstein, M.F.; McHugh, P.R.: Psychiatric syndromes in Huntington's disease. Adv. Neurol. *23:* 281–289 (1979).
Francis, A.F.: Familial basal ganglia calcification and schizophreniform psychosis. Br. J. Psychiat. *135:* 360–362 (1979).
Frankel, M.; Cummings, J.L.: Neuro-ophthalmic abnormalities in Gilles de la Tourette syndrome. Functional and anatomic implications. Neurology, Minneap. *34:* 359–361 (1984).
Freud, S.: A general introduction to psychoanalysis (Liverright, New York 1920).
Friede, R.L.; Magee, K.R.; Mack, E.W.: Idiopathic non-arteriosclerotic calcification of cerebral vessels. Archs Neurol. *5:* 279–286 (1961).
Garcia-Albea, E.; Franch, O.; Munoz, D.; Ricoy, J.R.: Brueghel's syndrome report of a case with postmortem studies. J. Neurol. Neurosurg. Psychiat. *44:* 437–440 (1981).
Garon, D.C.: Huntington's chorea and schizophrenia. Adv. Neurol. *1:* 729–734 (1973).
Gerlach, J.; Reisby, N.; Randrup.: Dopaminergic hypersensitivity and cholinergic hypofunction in the pathophysiology of tardive dyskinesia. Psychopharmacologia *34:* 21–35 (1974).
Golden, G.S.: The effect of central nervous system stimulants on Tourette syndrome. Ann. Neurol. *2:* 69–70 (1977).
Greenfield, J.G.; Bosanquet, F.D.: The brain-stem lesions in parkinsonism. J. Neurol. Neurosurg. Psychiat. *16:* 213–226 (1953).
Gysin, W.M.; Cooke, E.T.: Unusual mental symptoms in a case of hepatolenticular degeneration. Dis. nerv. Syst. *28:* 305–309 (1950).
Hamilton, M. Fish's schizophrenia; 3rd ed. (Wright PSG, Boston 1984).
Hoehn-Saric, R.: Neurotransmitters in anxiety. Archs gen. Psychiat. *39:* 735–742 (1982).
Hohman, L.B.: Epidemic encephalitis (lethargic encephalitis). Archs Neurol. Psychiat. *6:* 295–333 (1921).
Horn, S.: Some psychological factors in parkinsonism. J. Neurol. Neurosurg. Psychiat. *37:* 27–31 (1974).
Huntington, G.: On chorea. Med. Surg. Rep. *26:* 317–321 (1872).
Jackson, J.A.; Free, G.B.M.; Pike, H.V.: The psychic manifestations in paralysis agitans. Archs Neurol. Psychiat. *10:* 680–684 (1923).
Jackson, J.A.; Immerman, S.L.: A case of pseudosclerosis associated with a psychosis. J. nerv. ment. Dis. *49:* 5–13 (1919).
Jackson, J.A.; Jankovic, J.; Ford, J.: Progressive supranuclear palsy: clinical features and response to treatment in 16 patients. Ann. Neurol. *13:* 273–278 (1923).

Janati, A.; Appel, A.R.: Psychiatric aspects of progressive supranuclear palsy. J. nerv. ment. Dis. *172:* 85–89 (1984).

Jankovic, J.; Ford, J.: Blepharospasm and orofacial-cervical dystonia. Clinical and pharmacological findings in 100 patients. Ann. Neurol. *13:* 403–411 (1983).

Javoy-Agid, F.; Agid, Y.: Is the mesocortical dopaminergic system involved in Parkinson disease? Neurology, Minneap. *30:* 1326–1330 (1980).

Jelliffe, S.E.: Oculogyric crises as compulsion phenomena in post-encephalitis: their occurrence, phenomenology, and meaning. J. nerv. ment. Dis. *69:* 59–68, 165–184, 278–297, 415–426, 531–551, 666–679 (1929).

Jeste, D.V.; Wyatt, R.J.: Understanding and treating tardive dyskinesia (Guilford Press, New York 1982).

Kalamboukis, Z.; Molling, P.: Symmetrical calcification of the brain in the predominance in the basal ganglia and cerebellum. J. neuropath. exp. Neurol. *21:* 364–371 (1962).

Kasanin, J.; Crank, R.P.: A case of extensive calcification in the brain. Archs Neurol. Psychiat. *34:* 164–178 (1935).

Kemp, J.M.; Powell, T.P.S.: The cortico-striate projection in the monkey, Brain *93:* 525–546 (1970).

Klawans, H.L.; Falk, D.K.; Nausieda, P.A.; Weiner, W.J.: Gilles de la Tourette syndrome after long-term chlorpromazine therapy. Neurology, Minneap. *28:* 1064–1068 (1978).

Korenyi, C.; Whittier, J.R.; Conchado, D.: Stress in Huntington's disease (chorea). Dis. nerv. Syst. *33:* 339–344 (1972).

Kvale, J.N.: Amitriptyline in the management of progressive supranuclear palsy. Archs Neurol. *39:* 387–388 (1982).

Leff, J.P.; Isaacs, A.D.: Psychiatric examination in clinical practice (Blackwell, London 1981).

Laitenen, L.: Desipramine in treatment of Parkinson's disease. Acta neurol. scand. *45:* 109–113 (1969).

Lance, J.W.; McLeod, J.G.: A physiological approach to clinical neurology (Butterworths, Boston 1981).

Langston, J.W.; Forno, L.S.: The hypothalamus in Parkinson disease. Ann. Neurol. *3:* 129–133 (1978).

Lebensohn, F.M.; Jenkins, R.B.: Improvement of parkinsonism in depressed patients treated with ECT. Am. J. Psychiat. *132:* 283–285 (1975).

Marsden, C.D.: Blepharospasm-oromandibular dystonia syndrome (Brueghel's syndrome). J. Neurol. Neurosurg. Psychiat. *39:* 1204–1209 (1976).

Marsden, C.D.; Owen, D.A.L.: Mechanisms underlying emotional variation in parkinsonian tremor. Neurology, Minneap. *17:* 711–715 (1967).

Marsden, C.D.; Tarsey, D.; Baldessarini, R.J.: Spontaneous and drug-induced movement disorders in psychotic patients; in Benson, Blumer, Psychiatric aspects of neurologic disease, pp. 219–265 (Grune & Stratton, New York 1975).

McAlpine, D.: The pathology of the parkinsonian syndrome following encephalitis lethargica, with a note on the occurrence of calcification in this disease. Brain *46:* 255–280 (1923).

McHugh, P.R.; Folstein, M.F.: Psychiatric syndromes of Huntington's chorea: a clinical and phenomenologic study; in Benson, Blumer, Psychiatric aspects of neurologic disease, pp. 267–285 (Grune & Stratton, New York 1975).

Meninger, K.A.: Influenza and schizophrenia. Am. J. Psychiat. *82:* 469–529 (1926).

Messifia, F.S.; Knopp, W.; Vanecko, S.; O'Brien, V.; Corson, S.A.: Haloperidol therapy in Tourette's syndrome: neurophysiological, biochemical and behavioral correlates. Life Sci. *10:* 449–457 (1971).

Mindham, R.H.S.: Psychiatric symptoms in Parkinsonism. J. Neurol. Neurosurg. Psychiat. *33:* 188–191 (1970).

Mindham, R.H.S.; Marsden, C.D.; Parkes, J.D.: Psychiatric symptoms during L-dopa therapy for Parkinson's disease and their relationship to physical disability. Psychol. Med. *6:* 23–33 (1976).

Mishra, R.K.; Demirjian, C.; Katzman, R.; Makman, M.H.: A dopamine-sensitive adenylate cyclase in anterior limbic cortex and mesolimbic region of primate brain. Brain Res. *96:* 395–399 (1975).

Montgomery, M.A.; Clayton, P.J; Friedhoff, A.J.: Psychiatric illness in Tourette syndrome patients and first-degree relatives; in Friedhoff, Chase, Gilles de la Tourette syndrome, pp. 335–339 (Raven Press, New York 1982).

Morphew, J.A.; Sim, M.: Gilles de la Tourette's syndrome. A clinical and psychopathological study. Br. J. med. Psychol. *42:* 293–301 (1969).

Nauta, W.J.H.: Limbic innervation of the striatum; in Friedhoff, Chase, Gilles de la Tourette syndrome, pp. 41–47 (Raven Press, New York 1982).

Nauta, W.J.H.; Domesick, V.P.: Crossroads of limbic and striatal circuitry: hypothalamo-nigral connections; in Livingston, Hornykiewicz, Limbic mechanisms, pp. 75–93 (Plenum Press, New York 1978).

Nee, L.E.; Caine, E.D.; Polinski, R.J.; Eldridge, R.; Ebert, M.H.: Gilles de la Tourette syndrome. Clinical and family study of 50 cases. Ann. Neurol. *7:* 41–49 (1980).

Nee, L.E.; Polinsky, R.J.; Ebert, M.H.: Tourette Syndrome: clinical and family studies; in Friedhoff, Chase, Gilles de la Tourette syndrome, pp. 291–295 (Raven Press, New York 1982).

Neumann, M.A.: Iron and calcium dysmetabolism in the brain. J. Neuropath. exp. Neurol. *22:* 148–163 (1963).

Obeso, J.A.; Rothwell, J.C.; Marsden, C.D.: Simple tics in Gilles de la Tourette syndrome are not prefaced by a normal premovement EEG potential. J. Neurol. Neurosurg. Psychiat. *44:* 735–738 (1981).

Pandey, R.S.; Sreenivas, K.N.; Patil, N.M.; Swany, N.S.: Dopamine B-hydroxylase inhibition in a patient with Wilson's disease and manic symptoms. Am. J. Psychiat. *138:* 1628–1629 (1981).

Price, K.S.; Farley, I.J.; Hornykiewicz, O.: Neurochemistry of Parkinson's disease: relation between striatal and limbic dopamine. Adv. Biochem. Psychopharm. *17:* 293–300 (1978).

Pulst, S.-M.; Walshe, T.M.; Romero, J.A.: Carbon monoxide poisoning with features of Gilles de la Tourette's syndrome. Archs Neurol. *40:* 443–444 (1983).

Richards, F.II; Cooper, M.R.; Pearce, L.A.; Cowan, R.J.; Spurr, C.L.: Familial spinocerebellar degeneration, hemolytic anemia, and glutathion deficiency. Archs intern Med. *134:* 534–537 (1974).

Riley, A.H.: Epidemic encephalitis. Archs Neurol. Psychiat. *24:* 574–604 (1930).

Robins, A.H.: Depression in patients with parkinsonism. Br. J. Psychiat. *128:* 141–145 (1976).

Rosenbaum, D.: Psychosis with Huntington's chorea. Psychiat. Q. *15:* 93–99 (1941).
Sandy, W.C.: The association of neuro-psychiatric conditions with influenza in the epidemic of 1918. Archs Neurol. Psychiat. *4:* 171–181 (1920).
Scheinberg, I.H.; Steinlieb, I.: Wilson's disease (Saunders, Philadelphia 1984).
Schildkraut, J.J.: Neuropsychopharmacology and the affective disorders (Little, Brown, Boston 1970).
Schwab, R.S.; Zieper, I.: Effects of mood, motivation, stress and alertness on the performance in Parkinson's disease. Psychiatria Neurol., Basel *150:* 345–357 (1965).
Shapiro, A.K.; Shapiro, E.S.; Bruun, R.D.; Sweet, R.D.: Gilles de la Tourette syndrome (Raven Press, New York 1978).
Shephard, M.: Report of a family suffering from Friedreich's disease, muscular atrophy, and schizophrenia. J. Neurol. neurosurg. Psychiat. *18:* 297–304 (1955).
Shoulson, I.: Huntington disease: functional capacities in patients treated with neuroleptic and antidepressant drugs. Neurology, Minneap. *31:* 1333–1335 (1981).
Singer, H.S.: Tics and Tourette syndrome. Johns Hopkins med. J. *151:* 30–35 (1982).
Singer, H.S.; Butler, I.J.; Tune, L.E.; Seifert, W.E., Jr.; Coyle, J.T.: Dopaminergic dysfunction in Tourette syndrome. Ann. Neurol. *12:* 361–366 (1982).
Snyder, S.H.: Catecholamines, serotonin, and histamine; in Siegel, Albers, Katzman, Agranoff, Basic neurochemistry, pp. 203–217 (Little, Brown, Boston 1976).
Steele, J.C.: Progressive supranuclear palsy. Brain *95:* 693–704 (1972).
Steele, J.C.; Richardson, J.C.; Olszewski, J.: Progressive supranuclear palsy. Archs Neurol. *10:* 333–359 (1964).
Strang, R.R.: Imipramine in treatment of Parkinsonism: a double-blind placebo study. Br. med. J. *ii:* 33–34 (1965).
Sweeney, D.; Pickar, D.; Redmond, D.E., Jr.; Maas, J.: Noradrenergic and dopaminergic mechanisms in Gilles de la Tourette syndrome. Lancet *i:* 872 (1978).
Tarsy, D.; Baldessarini, R.J.: The pathophysiologic basis of tardive dyskinesia. Biol. Psychiat. *12:* 431–450 (1977).
Taylor, M.A.; Abrams, R.: Catatonia. Archs gen. Psychiat. *34:* 1223–1225 (1977).
Tolosa, E.S.: Clinical features of Meige's disease (idiopathic orofacial dystonia). Archs Neurol. *38:* 147–151 (1981).
Tolosa, E.S.; Klawans, H.L.: Meige's disease. A clinical form of facial convulsion, bilateral and medial. Archs Neurol. *36:* 635–637 (1979).
Tolosa, E.S.; Lai, C.-W.: Meige disease: striatal dopaminergic preponderance. Neurology, Minneap. *29:* 1126–1130 (1979).
Stevens, J.R.: Neuropathology of schizophrenia. Archs gen. Psychiat. *39:* 1131–1139 (1982).
Ungerstedt, U.: Stereotaxic mapping of the monoamine pathways in the rat brain. Acta physiol. scand., suppl. *367:* pp. 1–48 (1971).
Warburton, J.W.: Depressive symptoms in parkinson patients referred for thalomotomy. J. Neurol. Neurosurg. Psychiat. *30:* 368–370 (1967).
Weiner, W.J.; Werner, T.R.: Mania-induced remission of tardive dyskinesia in manic-depressive illness. Ann. Neurol. *12:* 229–230 (1982).
Whittier, J.; Haydu, G.; Crawford, J.: Effect of imipramine (Tofranil) on depression and hypokinesia in Huntington's disease. Am. J. Psychiat. *79:* 118 (1961).
Wohlfart, G.; Ingvar, D.H.; Hellberg, A.-M.: Compulsory shouting (Benedek's 'Klazomania') associated with oculogyric spasms in chronic epidemic encephalitis. Acta psychiat. scand. *36:* 369–377 (1961).

Yakovlev, P.I.: The central 'paradox' of Parkinson's disease. J. Neurosurg. suppl., part II, pp. 292–300 (1966).
Yarden, P.E.; Discipio, W.J.: Abnormal movements and prognosis in schizophrenia. Am. J. Psychiat. *128:* 317–323 (1971).

J.L. Cummings, MD, Neurobehavior Unit, West Los Angeles VAMC
(Brentwood Division), Los Angeles, CA 90073 (USA)

7. Psychosomatic Aspects of Epilepsy

Michael R. Trimble

The National Hospitals and Department of Neuropsychiatry, Institute of Neurology, University of London, UK

Introduction

Epilepsy is defined clinically as the liability to recurrent seizures during which abnormal electrical activity is recorded on an electroencephalogram. As such, it is a common human affliction, it occurs in approximately 0.5% of the population in the UK and is associated with considerable morbidity and some mortality. Being primarily a disorder which starts in childhood, its prognosis is dependent upon the age at which seizures begin, the underlying aetiology for the seizures, the extent of any associated brain damage, and the success or failure of treating seizures. The latter usually implies control by anticonvulsant medications, and it is now recognised that prolonged administration of these brings with it further morbidity, some of which have direct bearing on the ultimate psychiatric sequelae of epilepsy [*Trimble and Reynolds,* 1976]. Prior to discussion of the psychosomatic aspects of epilepsy, a brief introduction to the epileptic process, its causes, classification and treatment will be considered.

Epilepsy

The ultimate electrophysiological abnormality in an epileptic seizure is excessive electrical activity in neurones within the central nervous system provoking disorganisation of CNS function. Some of the underlying aetiologies are shown in table I, but it should be recognised that in many cases no clearly defined pathology is discerned, the type of epilepsy then being referred to as idiopathic.

Table I. Some causes of epilepsy

Metabolic causes	hypoglycaemia, hypomagnesaemia, fluid and electrolyte disturbances, acute intermittent porphyria, aminoacid disorders
Trauma	head injuries, especially penetrating wounds and birth injuries
Neurological causes	tumours, cerebrovascular accidents, degenerative and storgage disorders, demyelinating diseases, Sturge-Weber and other malformations, tuberose-sclerosis, infections, e.g., cytomegalovirus, toxoplamosis, meningitis, cysticercosis, syphilis
Drug withdrawal	especially alcohol and the barbiturates
Vitamin deficiency	pyridoxine
Poisons	lead, strychnine
Temperature	fever

The present classification of the epilepsies recognises two main categories, namely generalised epilepsy, in which the electroencephalographic discharge is generalised from the onset, and arises bilaterally, and partial epilepsies which are seen to originate from a focus in one or other hemisphere. Generally, the partial epilepsies are regarded as being the result of focal pathology, and a common form of partial epilepsy is that arising from the temporal lobes which has been referred to as temporal lobe epilepsy. The generalised epilepsies are further subdivided into so-called primary generalised epilepsy in which a genetic background is often clear, and secondary generalised epilepsy where there is evidence of brain damage, often of a diffuse nature, and usually acquired early in life.

In the clinic or on the ward what is usually observed in a patient with epilepsy is the seizure, namely the main clinical manifestation of the condition. Classification of the seizures has been more successful than classification of epilepsy per se, and an abbreviated classification of the seizures as recognised by the International League Against Epilepsy [*Gastaut*, 1969] is shown in table II. Again these are broadly divided into two main categories, namely partial seizures which begin locally and the generalised seizures which are bilaterally symmetrical from the onset. Partial seizures are further subdivided into various categories, the commonest being partial seizures with complex symptomatology, reminiscent of the older term psychomotor seizure. In these attacks, patients have alteration of higher

Table II. Classification of the seizures

Partial seizures	A simple or elementary	motor
		sensory
		autonomic
		compound
	B complex	impaired consciousness
		cognitive symptoms
		affective symptoms
		psychosensory symptoms
		compound
	C secondary generalised	
Generalized seizures		absences
		simple
		complex
		myoclonic
		infantile spasms
		clonic seizures
		tonic seizures
		tonic-clonic seizures
		atonic seizures
		akinetic seizures
Unilateral seizures		
Unclassified seizures		

cognitive function and impairment of consciousness as a necessary component of the seizure. As will be noted later, it is patients that have these attacks, which usually arise from the temporal lobes and form part of temporal lobe epilepsy, that much of the recent interest in psychiatric links in epilepsy have focused on.

Generalised seizures cover a variety of attacks including absence (petit mal) seizures, myoclonic seizures, tonic-clonic seizures (grand mal attacks) and atonic and akinetic seizures.

The importance of careful delineation of seizure type in the assessment of epilepsy is that effective treatments are now available for many patients with epilepsy providing that certain principles are followed. First, certain anticonvulsants are only effective in certain seizures. A list of some anticonvulsants currently in use are shown in table III. It is important to emphasise that ethosuximide is only of value in generalised absence seizures, and that neither phenytoin nor carbamazepine are helpful in the

Table III. Some anticonvulsant drugs in current use

Name	Half-life, h	Recommended serum levels, μmol/l	Indications
Carbamazepine (Tegretol)	8–45	16–40	generalized seizures; simple or complex partial seizures
Clobazam (Frisium)			secondary generalised; complex or simple partial seizures
Clonazepam (Rivotril)	20–40	–	myoclonic epilepsy
Ethosuximide (Zarontin)	30–100	300–700	'petit mal' epilepsy
Phenobarbitone	36 (children)	60–180	generalized or simple partial seizures
Phenytoin (Epanutin)	–	40–100	generalized seizures: simple or complex partial seizures
Primidone (Mysoline)	3–12	–	generalized: complex or simple partial seizures
Sodium valproate (Epilim)	10–15	–	'Petit mal': generalized seizures: myoclonic epilepsy; simple or complex partial seizures
Sulthiamine (Ospolot)	–	–	complex partial seizures

management of these attacks. Patients with partial seizures tend to respond better to carbamazepine, while those with generalised seizures are more commonly managed with sodium valproate or phenytoin. Phenobarbitone has been less favoured in recent years because of the known incidence of behavioural side effects it provokes. Primidone too is problematic since this drug is partly metabolised to phenobarbitone.

The second principle with regards to treatment of epilepsy is that where possible one anticonvulsant (monotherapy) should be used rather than two or more. *Reynolds and Shorvon* [1981] have convincingly demonstrated that 80–85% of adolescent or adult new out-patients may be controlled on single drug therapy and other studies indicate that the addition of a second drug is rarely beneficial from the point of view of control of seizures [*Schmidt* 1983]. Even patients with chronic epilepsy who are on polytherapy may benefit by judicious rationalisation of therapy, which, moreover, may result in not only improvement of seizure frequency but also improvement in cognitive function, mood and behaviour [Milano Collaborative Group, 1977; *Thompson and Trimble,* 1982].

The third principle of treatment is the utilisation of serum level monitoring particularly in patients not responding to therapy. While many patients may be controlled on a small dose of medication, good treatment emphasises monitoring of serum levels where there is question about patient compliance, where there is a possibility of toxicity from the anticonvulsant drug, or where, in spite of apparently good doses of drugs, the patient is persisting to have seizures.

Psychosomatic Aspects of Epilepsy

While it is common knowledge amongst physicians and amongst patients that stress is somehow related to seizures, often this linkage is merely tacitly assumed and no further discussed. History however is replete with comments on the associations and even postulated pathophysiologies. *Willis,* for example, in his Oxford lectures dating back to the 17th century, noted that epilepsy was caused by vitriolic humours, and had antecedent causes. He quoted 'anything that tended to agitate ..., for example anger, sudden passions, terror, joy, intemperance, drunkenness, immoderate excerise ...' [*Dewhurst,* 1980]. This one psychosomatic link with epilepsy has, however, been overshadowed by another, namely the association of personality and epilepsy, and in particular the concept that patients with certain personality profiles may be prone to develop epileptic seizures.

The Epileptic Personality

The literature on personality changes in epilepsy goes back to ancient times [*Guerrant* et al., 1962]. The changes regarding this concept as outlined by *Guerrant* and co-workers are shown in table IV. Thus, in the last century, the very fact that patients had epilepsy was seen to be enough to lead to association with an alteration and deterioration of personality, ideas being interlinked with moral degeneration and hereditary predisposition. In the early part of this century, however, a change in thinking was noted. The epilepsy itself and associated behavioural or personality changes were thus seen as secondary to some underlying third principle which was common to both. One of the potential uniting factors was the personality structure. These earlier views were then refuted by the writ-

Table IV. History of personality changes in epilepsy [from *Guerrant* et al., 1962]

Period of epileptic deterioration	–1900
Period of epileptic character	1900–1930
Period of normality	1930–
Period of psychomotor peculiarity	1930–

ings of authors such as *Lennox* [1944] who commented that most patients with epilepsy did not show typical or special personality traits, and suggested that patients with epilepsy were as normal as other people, with the exception that changes of personality could be provoked on account of recurrent brain damage, uncontrolled seizures, chronic anticonvulsant drug ingestion and psychosocial problems that were a consequence of having epilepsy.

The development of the electroencephalogram in the 1940s and 1950s led to the view that certain patients with a particular form of epilepsy, namely temporal lobe epilepsy, were more prone to the development of psychiatric disturbances than those with generalised epilepsies. These suggestions arose at the same time that authors such as *Papez* [1937] and *MacLean* [1970] were developing the concept of the limbic system, and its role in the elaboration of emotional experiences. Temporal lobe epilepsy was seen as a natural model of a limbic system disturbance in man, and its behavioural consequences thus became an important area of clinical research.

At the present time there is considerable argument as to whether or not patients with different forms of epilepsy display differing types of personality disturbance [*Trimble*, 1983]. However, many of the arguments do not take into account the differing historical view points with regards to the relationship of epilepsy and personality, and do not clearly define at least two, namely the earlier concept that patients with certain personalities may be prone to the development of seizures, and the more recently stated hypothesis that it is patients with temporal lobe epilepsy who, on account of the organic changes within the temporal lobes develop secondary personality changes that may have some specificity related to the site of the abnormality in the brain. It is the former view point which is of most interest to psychosomatic medicine.

The concept of the epileptic constitution was hinted at in the writings of *Fere* [1890] who believed that the character and manner of patients with epilepsy arouse suspicion of the disease long before the appearance of convulsions.

Charcot, who, working at Salpêtrière in Paris, was one of the last neurologists to take the neuroses seriously as a research interest, was concerned with both somatic and psychological mechanisms in the development of symptoms, and was instrumental in educating both *Freud* and *Janet. Janet* was particularly interested in the relationship of personality to symptoms, and held the view that in certain patients, particularly those prone to hysteria, the central nervous system was somehow weak. Epilepsy and hysteria were closely linked in the minds of many authors at that time, particularly in France, and such terms as hysteroepilepsy are to be found in the literature. *Janet* [1929] thought that the epileptic attack represented a lowering of psychic tension linking together in his theories epilepsy, hysteria and psychaesthenia. *Freud* more clearly drew relationships between the constitution, epileptic and hysterical convulsions as noted in the following quotation:

> 'In infants apart from the respiratory action of screaming affects only produce and find expression in unco-ordinated contractions of the muscles of this primitive kind – in arching the body and kicking about. As development proceeds the musculature passes more and more under the control of the power of co-ordination and the will, but the opisthotonus which represents the maximum of motor effort of the total somatic musculature and the clonic movements of the kicking and thrashing about persist throughout life as a form of reaction for the maximal excitation of the brain – for the purely physical excitation in epileptic attacks as well as for the discharge of maximal affects in the shape of more or less epileptoid convulsions.'

Freud further elucidated mechanisms with regards to epilepsy with his psychological study of the life and character of Dostoevski [*Freud*, 1929]. *Freud* linked his epilepsy to the Oedipus complex, suggesting its content as a punishment for fantasied parricide and noted how the seizures satisfy guilt through masochism. *Fenichel* [1931] also reflected on the narcissistic regression in epilepsy, the energy tension in the brain being an expression of sadistic impulses. *Stekel* [1924] described the epileptic seizure as an escape from an unbearable situation, the traumatic events that form the point of crystallization often residing in childhood events. *Kardiner* [1932] developed further the theme of trauma in epilepsy suggesting that the traumatic neurosis established the basic patterns upon which the epileptic reaction was based, and emphasising the importance of genital development for determining the clinical character of the epilepsy.

Pierce-Clark [1929] was one of the more persistent writers of this era and he attempted to present a psychobiological theory of epilepsy implicating Freudian psychodynamics to explain certain types of epilepsy. He pointed out that in many cases no neuropathological disorder can be demonstrated, and from his own studies of epileptic patients he was able to discern certain patterns of developmental traits which were seen prior to the onset of the epilepsy. His suggestion echoed that of *Freud,* namely that the fit served as an unconscious gratification for the libido, thus, 'the epileptic reaction places itself at the disposal of the neurosis, the essence of which is to get rid by somatic means, of masses of stimulae which it can not deal with psychically'. Thus, in both epilepsy and in the neurosis, infantile motives and the inadequate development of the individuals affects and instincts led to the later development of the symptoms. This was referring mainly to idiopathic generalised seizures, and indeed on a discussion of 'essential epilepsy', *Lehrman* [1925] made a similar point. He said 'the symptoms of psychoneurosis, psychosis, and essential (psychogenic) epilepsy, indicate not only the intensity of the unconscious strivings, but the necessity of the manner and degree of withdrawal from reality. Thus, a partial withdrawal is seen in the psychoneurosis, a complete withdrawal is seen in the psychosis, and a sudden withdrawal is seen in epilepsy.'

Billings [1946] referred to the epileptic attack as a psychobiological reaction in certain persons with a predisposition for it, and *Jelliffe and White* [1929] considered the epileptic seizures as 'the flight into unconsciousness' which occurred maximally at times of stress. *Rows and Bond* [1926] felt that a disturbance of the emotional life was found in every epileptic patient, considering the disease a functional psychiatric illness, the somatic manifestations of which are preceeded by complex psychic activity.

Intermingled with these ideas were to be found concepts such as the 'epileptoid' character, and of epileptic equivalents, which then became confused with the developing concept of psychomotor epilepsy and the notion of 'psychomotor personality change' secondary to temporal lobe lesions [*Hill,* 1981]. *Bratz and Leubuscher* [1907] had defined affect epilepsy which they were able to distinguish from 'real epilepsy', and which was characterised by seizures induced by psychological excitation. These attacks were accompanied by loss of consciousness, dizziness, hallucinations, and rage attacks, although no dementia was observed in the progression of the disorder. They thought this was a genetically determined illness which was not hysterical, and commented that *Oppenheim* had also observed similar attacks following such stress in psychaesthenic individuals.

Rockwell et al. [1947] discussed epileptoid psychopathological reactions. These comprised of episodes with a well-designed onset and termination which included attacks of unmotivated irritability accompanied by resentment, suspiciousness and ideas of reference. These were accompanied by marked thinking disorders and a degree of confusion, sometimes associated with an alteration of the sense of reality. Linking this to epilepsy the authors comment: 'The role of psychodynamic factors, including that of emotions, must be considered from the same point of view in epileptoid as in epileptic disorders.' They studied 11 patients fulfilling these criteria, all of whom had abnormal electroencephalograms (three were paroxysmal, two of them showing 'abortive spike and dome complexes') with the Rorschach test. The pattern of responses was the same as that seen in epileptic patients.

That such ideas were maintained well in this century is exemplified by *Gordin* who, as late as 1953, wrote a thesis entitled: 'The epileptic cramp attack as a psychosomatic reaction.' He emphasised that the constant association noted by several eminent authors of fits, resembling major tonic-clonic attacks, seen in hysterics, psychoaesthenic and psychopathic personalities proved that hysterical attacks and epileptic seizures were more related than they had hitherto been considered [p. 10]. He felt that from the point of view of brain function, the epileptic is classified with these personality types as 'vegetatively stigmatized', emphasising a common type of reaction.

Much of this early work implying characterological predisposition in patients who later develop epilepsy has now been discredited. At the present time it is reasonable to say that the concept of the epileptic personality is not accepted by the majority of physicians who deal with epilepsy and many of these earlier investigations are likely to remain in the history books. As discussed below, however, a recrudescence of some of these ideas is occurring with new discoveries which relate to the biochemistry of both epilepsy and psychiatry.

The Relationship of Stress to Seizure Precipitation

Amongst those of the last century who clearly acknowledged this relationship was *Hughlings Jackson*. Writing in an era prior to *Freud,* for him it was not the psychological content of an emotion which was relevant, but the general change in the body which occurred with strong emotions that could lead to a discharge of unstable nerve cells. The discussion on 'affect epilepsy' above indicates that such episodes were recognised by other physicians and that there did exist patients whose epileptic seizures were provoked by strong emotions. This further led to the concept of the seizure having some protective value for the patient, in the way of homeostasis, somehow relieving excessive emotion and restoring harmony. *Aring* et al. [1947] after describing some case histories in which 'accumulated rage' appeared to disperse following a grand mal seizure, wrote: 'The intense rage induced a general psychosomatic dysequilibrium, restitution of equilibrium followed the massive motor discharge.' He was keen to point out that the seizures represented an economical use of readily available pathways through which tension could be reduced and equilibrium re-established, but went on to say: 'this is not evidence for a primary psychogenesis of epilepsy, but does support the concept that epileptic phenomena result from the activation of primitive neural pathways when homeostasis is disturbed by physiological or emotional stress.' *Fremont-Smith* [1934] studied 42 unselected 'private patients' with generalised convulsions, noting in 31 a direct relation between emotion and one or more seizures. The emotions were usually fear, guilt or frustration, and in several cases attacks were precipitated by discussion of emotional problems. With the development of the electroencephalogram several authors attempted to explore further the changes in electrical activity in the central nervous system of patients with epilepsy during stressful events. *Stevens* [1958] studied the effects of 'strong emotional stimuli' on the electroencephalogram of 30 patients with generalised and partial seizures. During a stress interview the investigator directed a series of questions, criticisms, accusations, and, finally, laudatory comments and apologies to the subject while the EEG recording continued. She noted that 75% of patients with psychomotor epilepsy developed abnormal responses, in many these not being recorded on routine records. Altogether 20 patients demonstrated abnormal recordings in response to stress, 9 showing a clear cut exaggeration of spiking or paroxysmal activity. In 11 patients pathological epileptiform responses were elicited which had not been seen using conventional activation procedures.

Groethuysen et al. [1957] discussed the case history of a patient with depth electroencephalographic recordings, the electrodes being placed in some limbic system structures. Items of increasing emotional impact were presented to the patient and following an emotionally charged interpretation, changes were noted on the electrodes, particularly in the region of the left amygdala, with the slow development of a seizure discharge and a post-ictal slow wave focus. The interesting and unusual thing about this case history was that although the patient was awaiting surgery for a schizophrenia-like illness, and convulsions were not seen in the 7 days of observation following implantation of the electrodes prior to the experiment, the patient had not had a recorded convulsive seizure for 40 years prior to the structured interview.

Berkhout et al. [1969] carried out a spectral analysis of the electroencephalogram in 14 male volunteers between the ages of 18 and 22 who were given 20 questions that covered a variety of personal and ethical topics, ranging from the embarrassing or offensive to the innocuous. The degree of stress they suffered was measured by assessing autonomic arousal, and they found that high stress epocs were characterised by 'a distinct narrowing of the temporo-parietal theta band width, a similar narrowing of the occipital alpha band width, and a 70% increase in fronto-temporal beta intensity'. Although this was not an investigation in epileptic patients, it emphasised the effect of stress on electroencephalographic patterns in the healthy brain.

Using the more sophisticated prolonged ambulatory monitoring of the electroencephalogram, *Stores and Lwin* [1981] collected recordings from 28 children who suffered from absence seizures and recorded the children's activities throughout the day by means of diaries. In 5 cases they were able to note a peak occurrence of seizure activity that was associated with psychological or physiological factors recorded in the diaries including worry, boredom, drowsiness, physical activity, and hunger.

These data then provide some evidence that stressful psychological events alter EEG parameters and may in certain situations precipitate seizures especially in those that have pre-existing epilepsy. There are three important consequences of this: the first has regard to terminology, the second to treatment, and the third to mechanism.

It has long been recognised that epilepsy may be precipitated by a variety of environmental phenomena. Generally, these have been referred to as reflex epilepsies, and the subject has been reviewed by several authors [*Merlis*, 1974; *Fenwick*, 1981]. Most discussed are auditory or somatosensory evoked seizures, but there are clearly a group of patients who have attacks which are triggered by some specific mental activity. The correct term for these is probably psychogenic seizures [*Fenwick*, 1981] and the inappropriate use of 'psychogenic seizures' to refer to non-epileptic (hysterical) convulsions is to be depreciated. *Fenwick* [1981] divides psychogenic seizures into primary, those in which 'a direct act of will could precipitate a seizure', and secondary, namely those that are 'precipitated by a specific function of the mind without a deliberate intention on the part of the patient to precipitate a seizure, and without a clear evoking peripheral stimulus'. In the first group are patients who have learned that by carrying out a certain mental activity they could produce a seizure. In some patients concentration on an emotion, for example, sadness, may be sufficient [*Fenwick*, 1981].

The investigations and literature reviewed above, however, are not related to seeking such direct influences of the emotions on seizure events, but with a more difficult phenomena to clarify, namely the role of stress generally and heightened emotion in particular on the provokation of seizures. In fact, these kinds of events should not be included in the classification of reflex epilepsies, and the stress should be seen as one of several provoking factors which may exacerbate the tendency to recurrent seizures.

The fact that patients have seizures precipitated by stress leads to consideration of treatment. Again, there is considerable literature, mainly with anecdotal case records, of methods that have been used to inhibit seizures in patients with epilepsy, some of the literature on this, in particular with regards to behavior modification, being discussed by *Cobb* (chap. 8). The essential point of this is that there are patients who develop their own idiosyncratic techniques to inhibit seizures which include relaxation, or the deliberate carrying out of some mental or motor act. These provide important examples of the influence of psychological activity on somatic phenomena and they deserve further investigation than at the present time they have been given.

Mechanisms of Psychosomatic Links in Epilepsy

With regard to psychogenic seizures, both primary and secondary, it has been suggested that specific forms of mental activity are associated with the activation of neuronal circuits which, if themselves are epileptogenic, will lead to provocation of seizures [*Fenwick*, 1981]. However, the other associations discussed are not reflex, and the investigations, for example, of *Stevens* [1958], indicate a latency of several seconds to minutes between the emotional events and the onset of the attack. In other situations, stress is seen as an even more nebulous concept which patients experience, and which is associated with an increase in seizures although a direct one-to-one relationship is not envisaged. The early psychosomatic speculations of authors such as *Clarke* are discussed above. The discovery of the reticular activating system, and the observations of, for example, *Murphy and Gelhorn* [1945] that stimulation of the hypothalamus leads to seizure activity in a pharmacologically predisposed cortex suggests an interrelationship between subcortical activity and cortical structures, alteration of activity in the former leading to changes of seizure threshold in the latter. Some experimental evidence for this comes from the work of *Swinyard* et al. [1963], who stressed mice with intermittent foot shock and noted that this led to a lowering of the experimental seizure threshold. They speculated, however, that this was due to alteration of hormonal output from the adrenal medulla. Bringing to mind earlier concepts such as those of *Bratz and Leubuscher* [1907], *Lieberson* [1955] directly discussed the limbic system as being involved in reflex epilepsy. This area he felt could be sensitised by a real pathological process, and induced to discharge by stimuli with emotional significance. One could thus consider the existence of an 'affectogenic epilepsy'.

With regard to the more chronic stress that the patients with epilepsy find themselves facing, either on account of or inspite of their seizure disorder, we may seek further physiological explanations. *Fremont-Smith* [1934] suggested 'stimulation of the sympathetic nervous system by emotion'. *Friis and Lund* [1974] reviewed the case records of 1,250 patients with epilepsy and found 37 who suffered from what they referred to as stress convulsions. Interestingly, these patients often had a family history of epilepsy and in 4 out of 5 cases more than 1 'stress factor' seemed involved. Lack of sleep was found to be one of the commonest provoking factors, followed by bodily overexertion and emotional stress. Thus, since stress may lead to sleep disturbances this is a very acceptable and understandable mechanism for the provocation of seizures, and there are many reports in the literature showing the effect of sleep deprivation on seizures, both in animals and in man. For example, *Rodin* et al. [1962], using electroencephalographic records from healthy volunteers who had up to 120 h of sleep deprivation noted in some the appearance of high voltage diffuse paroxysmal activity most pronounced after 24–48 h of deprivation. In 2 subjects, light sensitivity developed and in another a major seizure followed provocation.

Another obvious relationship that emerges from these ideas is the link between depressive illness and epilepsy. Thus, depression is commonly found in epileptic patients [*Robertson and Trimble,* 1982], and sleep disorder is an early primary symptom of this. Although the mechanism of the

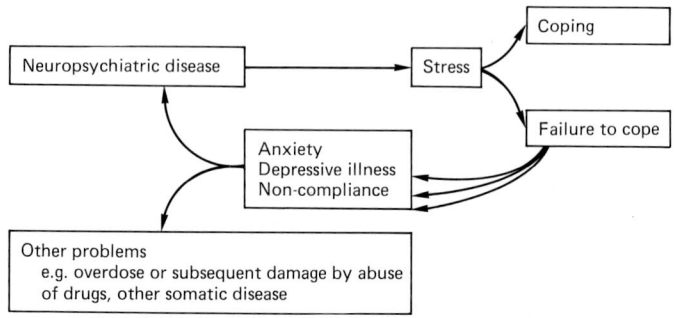

Fig. 1. Links between stress and neuropsychiatric illness.

sleep disorder in depressive illness is not clear, it is interesting that one of the biochemical underpinnings of depressive illness is thought to relate to disturbances of serotonin metabolism, and that sleep disorder is also interlinked with this neurotransmitter. Further, lowering serotonin in the central nervous system tends to decrease the threshold for seizures [*Chadwick* et al., 1975] and we therefore see three factors namely sleep disturbance, increased seizures, and depressive illness, all of which relate to serotonergic mechanisms, and all of which may be seen clinically in patients with epilepsy (fig. 1).

Neuropsychiatric illness itself brings about increased stress which may exacerbate the primary illness and lead to secondary complications. Some of these links are shown in figure 2 with special reference for epilepsy. Thus, it is widely acknowledged and accepted that patients with epilepsy have considerable social stigmatisation, and are markedly disadvantaged compared with many other patient groups. Not only is the threat of persistent loss of consciousness with potential embarrassment and loss of dignity and esteem demoralising, but there are the additional disadvantages educationally, emotionally and vocationally that the patient with epilepsy suffers. This starts in childhood in which, as *Williams* [1981] points out, the child with epilepsy does not 'feel' the stress, it simply biologically is 'there' in the family. The security of family unity is eroded: there is the loneliness of covert anxiety. It continues through adolescence and adulthood, permeating all lifes major events. As figure 2 indicates, adequate coping may be one outcome but frequently there is failure to cope and with this increasing psychiatric morbidity. Compliance with medication and the doctor's instructions tends to deteriorate, depressive symptoms may supervene with increasing seizure frequency and behaviour disturbances, overdoses, and further somatic damage.

The possible relationship between alteration of monoamine neurotransmitters and increased seizures is mentioned above, although other links could be postulated. For example, there is growing evidence that gamma-aminobutyric (GABA) may be involved in the regulation of the seizure threshold [*Meldrum*, 1978], which neurotransmitter may also be linked with affective disturbance with decreased GABA being noted in the CSF of some patients with depressive illness and GABA-ergic drugs showing antidepressant properties [*Morselli* et al., 1980]. A recent discovery has been the characterisation of benzodiazepine receptors within the central nervous system. Thus, benzodiazepines have enjoyed considerable use in recent years as anxiolytics but it is well recognised that they are also used in the management of epilepsy [*Trimble*, 1983]. Although their clinical use has been mainly confined to intravenous diazepam or clonazepam in status epilepticus, orally both nitrazepam and clonazepam have found use in the management of childhood epilepsies, particularly myoclonic epilepsies. More recently, the 1,5-benzodiazepine clobazam has found use as an anticonvulsant, being particularly beneficial in chronic intractable cases with complex partial seizures [*Allen* et al., 1982].

There thus seems to be a link between anxiety and epilepsy such that drugs which are anxiolytic are also anticonvulsant, and this seems to hinge around activity at the benzodiazepine-GABA receptor. Some of the more newly introduced benzodiazepine partial agonists confirm this relationship since compounds such as ethyl-β-carboline-3-carboxylate are proconvulsant and anxiogenic. Since anxiety is a principle manifestation of stress, and since benzodiazepine receptors are found all over the brain but concentrate particularly in certain regions, for example, the amydala of the limbic system, and since stress can provoke seizures or seizure activity in these limbic system structures, we have further important biochemical links to strengthen our understanding of the relationship between stress and epilepsy.

Conclusion

In this chapter, following a brief introduction to some of the clinical aspects of epilepsy two main psychosomatic links have been explored. In the first, now mainly of historical interest, the literature on epileptic personality is reviewed, particularly that which implies that epilepsy is in someway intimately related with personality variables. In the second half of the chapter the role that stress may play in the precipitation of seizures is further explored, and finally, some possible biological and chemical underpinnings for these relationships noted. It is hoped that as our understanding of brain structure and function increases and the links between the brain's behaviour and personality become clearer, that psychosomatic relationships in neuropsychiatric disease, in particular epilepsy, may be better understood and the subject of further scientific investigation.

References

Allen, J.W.; Oxley, J.; Robertson, M.M.; Trimble, M.R.; Richens, A; Jawad, S.S.M.: Clobazam as an adjunctive treatment in refractory epilepsy. Br. med. J. 286: 1246–1247 (1983).

Aring, C.D.; Lederer, H.D.; Rosenbaum, M.: The role of emotion in the causation of epilepsy. ARNMD 26: 561–572 (1947).

Berkhout, J.; Walter, D.O.; Adey, W.R.: Alterations of the human electroencephalogram induced by stressful verbal activity. Electroencephal. clin. Neurophysiol. 27: 457–469 (1969).

Billings, E.G.: Handbook of elementary psychobiology (Macmillan, New York 1946).

Bratz, H.; Leubuscher, H.: Die Affekt-Epilepsie, eine klinische, von der Echten Epilepsie abtrennbare Gruppe. Dt. med. Wschr. 33: 592–593 (1907).

Chadwick, D.; Jenner, P.; Reynolds, E.H.: Amines, anticonvulsants and epilepsy. Lancet i: 473–476 (1975).

Dewhurst, K.: Thomas Willis's Oxford lectures (Sandford Publications, Oxford 1980).

Fenichel, O.: Hysterie und Zwangsneurosen (Wien 1931).

Fenwick, P.: EEG studies; in Reynolds, Trimble, Epilepsy and psychiatry, pp. 242–263 (Churchill Livingstone, Edinburgh 1981).

Fere, M. (1890): Quoted by Pierce-Clarke (1920).

Fremont-Smith, F.: The influence of emotion in precipitating convulsions. Am. J. Psychiat. 13: 717–723 (1934).

Freud, S.: Dostoevski and parricide. Realist 1: (1929).

Friis, M.L.; Lund, M.: Stress convulsions. Archs Neurol. 31: 155–159 (1974).

Gastaut, H.: Clinical and electroencephalographic classification of epileptic seizures. Epilepsia, suppl. 10, pp. s2–s21 (1969).

Guerrant, J.; Anderson, W.W.; Fischer, A.; Weinstein, M.R.; Jaros, R.M.; Deskins, A.: Personality in epilepsy (Thomas, Springfield 1962).

Gordin, R.A.F.: The epileptic cramp attack as a psychosomatic reaction (Helsingfors 1953).

Groethuysen, U.C.; Robinson, D.B.; Haylett, C.H.; Estes, H.R.; Johnson, A.M.: Depth EEG recording of a seizure during a structured interview. Psychosom. Med. 19: 353–362 (1957).

Hill, D.: Historical review; in Reynolds, Trimble, Epilepsy and psychiatry, pp. 1–11 (Churchill-Livingstone, Edinburgh 1981).

Janet, P.: The major symptoms of hysteria (London 1929).
Jelliffe, S.E.; White, W.A.: Diseases of the nervous system (Lewis, London 1929).
Kardiner, A.: The bio-analysis of the epileptic reaction. Psychoanal. Q. *1:* 375–383 (1932).
Lehrman, P.R.: In discussion. Some psychological data regarding the interpretation of essential epilepsy. J. nerv. ment. Dis. *51:* 55 (1925).
Lennox, W.G.: Epilepsy; in Hunt, Handbook of personality and behaviour problems (Ronald Press, New York 1944).
Lieberson, W.T.: Emotional and psychological factors in epilepsy: physiological background. Am. J. Psychiat. *34:* 91–106 (1955).
MacLean: The triune brain, emotion of scientific basis; in The neurosciences second study programme, pp. 336–349 (Rockefellar University Press, New York 1970).
Meldrum, B.: Gaba and the search for new anticonvulsant drugs. Lancet *8084:* 304–306 (1978).
Merlis, J.K.: Reflex epilepsy; in Magnus, Lorentz De Haas, Handbook of clinical neurology, vol. 15, pp. 440–456 (North Holland Elsevier, Amsterdam 1974).
Milano Collaborative Group for Studies on Epilepsy: Long term intensive monitoring in the difficult patient; in Gardner, Janz Meinardi, Thorpe, Pippenger, Antiepileptic drug monitoring, Pitman, Tunbridge Wells, pp. 197–213 (1977).
Morselli, P.; Bossi, L.; Henry, J.; Zarifian, E.; Bartholini, G.: On the therapeutic action of SL 76002, a new GABA mimetic agent: preliminary observations in neuropsychiatric disorders. Brain Res. Bull. *5:* suppl. 2, pp. 411–414 (1980).
Murphy, J.P.; Gellhorn, E.: The influence of hypothalamic stimulation on cortically induced movements and on action potentials of the cortex. J. Neurophysiol: *8:* 341–364 (1945).
Papez, J.W.: A proposed mechanism of emotion. Archs Neurol. Psychiat. *38:* 725–743 (1937).
Pierce-Clark, L.: A psychological interpretation of essential epilepsy. Brain *43:* 38–49 (1929).
Reynolds, E.H.; Shorvon, S.: Monotherapy or polytherapy for epilepsy. Epilepsia *22:* 1–10 (1981).
Robertson, M.M.; Trimble, M.R.: Depressive illness in patients with epilepsy. A review. Epilepsia *24:* suppl. 2, pp. s109–s116 (1983).
Rockwell, F.V.; Sherfey, M.J.; Diethelm, O.: Epileptoid psychopathological reaction. ARNMD *26:* 573–585 (1947).
Rodin, E.A.; Luby E.D.; Gottlieb, J.S.: The EEG during prolonged experimental sleep deprivation. Electroencephal. clin. Neurophysiol. *14:* 544–551 (1962).
Rows, R.J.; Bond, W.E.: Epilepsy as a functional mental illness (H.K. Lewis, London 1926).
Schmidt, D.: Two antiepileptic drugs for intractable epilepsy with complex partial seizures. J. neurol. Neurosurg. Psychiat. *45:* 1119–1125 (1983).
Stekel, W.: Der epileptische Symptom-Complex; in Nervöse Angstzustände (Wien 1924).
Stevens, J.: Emotional activation of electroencephalogram in patients with convulsive disorders. J. nerv. ment. dis. *128:* 339–351 (1958).
Stores, G.; Lwin, R.: A study of factors associated with the occurrence of generalised seizure discharge in children with epilepsy using the Oxford Medilog System for ambulatory monitoring; in Dam, Gram, Penry, Advances in epileptology, pp. 421–422 (Raven Press, New York 1981).
Swinyard, E.A.; Miyahara, J.T.; Clarke, L.D.; Goodman, L.S.: The effects of experimen-

tally induced stress on pentylenetetrazol seizure threshold in mice. Psychopharmacologia 4: 345–353 (1963).
Thompson, P.J.; Trimble, M.R.: Anticonvulsant drugs and cognitive functions. Epilepsia 23: 531–544 (1982).
Trimble, M.R.: Interictal behaviour and temporal lobe epilepsy; in Pedley, Meldrum, Recent advances in epilepsy, vol. 1, pp. 211–229 (Churchill-Livingstone, Edinburgh 1983).
Trimble, M.R.: Benzodiazepines in epilepsy; in Trimble, Benzodiazepines divided, pp. 277–290 (Wiley, Chichester 1983).
Trimble, M.R.; Reynolds, E.H.: Anticonvulsant drugs and mental symptoms. A review. Psychol. Med. 6: 169–178 (1976).
Williams, D.: The emotions and epilepsy; in Reynolds, Trimble, Epilepsy and psychiatry, pp. 49–59 (Churchill-Livingstone, Edinburgh 1981).

Michael R. Trimble, MRCP, FRCPsych., Consultant Physician in Psychological Medicine, The National Hospitals, London WC1N 3BG (UK)

8. Behavioural Psychotherapy for Neurological Illness

John Cobb

Department of Psychiatry, St. George's Hospital, University of London, UK

Behavioural psychotherapy is a term that covers both a style of approach to clinical problems and a number of differentiated treatment techniques. Historically, it derives from the clinical application of findings in experimental psychology, particularly from research into learning theory. Present-day behavioural methods, however, have a much wider base. On the one hand, laboratory findings in cognitive psychology have provided an important stimulus in the development of new treatments. On the other hand, several behavioural methods have been derived pragmatically and await a satisfactory theoretical understanding. Since many readers may be unfamiliar with what actually goes on in the behavioural clinic, the first part of this chapter will be devoted to a brief description of the way a behavioural therapist approaches neurological problems and the various techniques used. This will be followed by a critical account of outcome research into those conditions in which there have been claims that behavioural treatment methods may be useful. These are epilepsy, migraine, tension headache, back pain, tics (including spasmodic torticollis and Gilles de la Tourette syndrome), writer's cramp, and defects resulting from brain damage.

The Behavioural Assessment

One of the cardinal features of the behavioural approach is that it is symptom orientated. Formerly, behaviourists were interested solely in overt behaviour, but now equal attention is paid to internal psychological 'behaviour', such as thoughts, attitudes, memories, perceptions and mood states which can only be observed indirectly. In assessing a patient with writer's cramp for example, the therapist will want to observe the symptom directly by asking the patient to attempt to write in front of him, noting carefully the sequence of muscle contraction and spasm which make writing difficult or impossible. Of equal importance will be the patient's attitude to the symptoms; the thoughts that flash through the mind at the first indication that writing is becoming difficult, and the increasing anxiety and frustration with which this is accompanied.

Symptom orientation focusses the therapist's attention in the here and now. Three aspects of this are of prime importance:

(1) *Cues or triggers.* A search is made for antecedent events which seem to be linked to onset of symptoms. One patient with writer's cramp for example developed her symptons only when she attempted to sign her name in a public place and when she felt she was being watched. Under scrutiny of the cashier, signature was impossible though she could sign without difficulty on a desk away from view. Similarly, the behavioural analysis of a case of reading epilepsy [*Forster* et al., 1969] showed that the content of the passage read was irrelevant. Seizures were provoked equally, whether reading passages of nonsense or exerpts from Shaw's 'Anthony and Cleopatry'. However, the reading had to be done out loud with lip movements, since reading silently without lip movements did not provoke fits. It is not always possible to obtain such clear cues, particularly in the first interview. However, symptoms which appear to the patient to come out of the blue, may be shown to be at least in part related to precipitating events. One of the functions of the 'Behavioural diary', which the patient is asked to fill in, between first and second appointments, is to aid in this process (table I).

A much more sophisticated experimental technique for identifying emotional triggers in epilepsy has been described by *Feldman and Paul* [1976]. Following initial interviews, individualised 'stressor tapes' were prepared. A number of different sources were used ranging from excerpts from films to audio or video readings of role played conversations between the patient and someone else, usually a family member or employer, likely to provoke strong emotional responses in the patient. These tapes were then presented in an orderly and systematic manner, fits being frequently triggered during this procedure which was videotaped. Replay in a sub-

Table 1. A specimen of a behavioural symptom diary designed for use by a patient suffering from tension headaches

Headache Diary

Please note all headaches that trouble you over the next week, preferably as they occur

Date	Time	Severity 0 — 10 (absent) (very severe)	Onset			Duration	Consequences (including methods of coping)
			place	activity	thoughts		

sequent session allowed the patient to see themselves having a fit and to discuss the events leading up to the seizure. This could bring about a heightened awareness of actual triggering circumstances and of interpersonal situations likely to precipitate seizures. Seizure cues included various conversations, spoken invectives, imagined concepts or fantasy, or incorrect perceptions of personal interaction.

(2) *Situations associated with symptoms.* Symptoms may be particularly likely to occur when patients are in certain places, in particular mood states or with certain other people. One epilepic patient recognised that most of her fits occurred when she was near a busy road and accompanied by her young children. Further enquiry revealed that in this situation she became frightened that she might have a fit, not because of the consequences to herself but because of what might happen to her children. Another example is given by an ingenious study, which examined the effect of the presence of a spouse on pain behaviour in a group of patients with chronic pain [*Block* et al., 1980]. In this study, patients were told that the assessment interview would be observed through a one-way screen either by the spouse or by a ward clerk. Previous assessment of the spouses had divided them into those who tended to show solicitous responses to their partner's pain and those who did not. The experimenter's prediction, based on operant learning theory, was that the patients with solicitous spouses would show more pain-related behaviour if the assessment were observed by the spouse than by the neutral observer and vice versa. The results confirmed these predictions. Again, the behavioural diary can be useful in revealing a previously unrecognised aspect of the problem. For example, an adolescent boy with Gilles de la Tourette syndrome was able to see from his diary that his tic and expletives were made worse when he was made anxious, either following a row with his father or else when he was trying to socialise with people he did not know well.

(3) *Consequences.* Occurrence of symptoms usually produces a reaction either in the patients themselves or in those they come in contact with. The patient with writer's cramp, for example, felt stupid and ashamed because of her symptoms and came to avoid public situations increasingly. The reaction of other family members was particularly important in the case of a middle-aged lady who complained of frequent severe and debilitating headaches. The behavioural analysis revealed that whenever she developed a headache she retired to her bedroom and was then treated by

her husband and 2 adolescent children 'like a queen'. In contrast when she was well, the family either ignored her or else made demands on her to do domestic chores.

Another aspect of this preliminary analysis, which is emphasised in a behavioural assessment concerns *quantification* and *self-monitoring*. Some symptoms such as pain and anxiety by their nature are variable in intensity and can easily be described on a 0–10 scale. Thus, an 'awful' headache becomes a headache which rates 8 on a severity scale. Measurement in this way allows a patient to track the course of a symptom over time and helps to increase awareness of those factors which increase or decrease its severity. It is also valuable to ask the patient to mark on the severity scale that point at which the symptom becomes unbearable, thus forcing some response such as taking a pill or retiring to bed. Further discussion may show that the cut off point that determines how intense a symptom can be endured depends not only on internal sensation, but also on the external situation. This is particularly important in the assessment of pain when, for example, the patient may well be much less distressed by the symptom when distracted than when sitting with nothing to do, or when lying in bed.

Three cognitive factors are of particular importance in the behavioural approach. First is the *patient's attitude to their own symptoms*. Does the patient believe that the symptoms are caused by some physical abnormality? If so, is this thought to be progressive and dangerous? Equally important is whether or not emotional factors are seen as playing a part. If so, are these in any way seen as being potentially under the patient's control. One patient with long-standing back pain firmly believed that 'pain is nature's way of warning you that you are damaging your body when you move'. For this reason she froze every time she felt a twinge of pain. The importance of her attitude was shown by subsequent events. After some discussion involving elementary anatomy, physiology and pathology, she came to accept that at least to some extent her discomfort and disability were the result of weakness and spasm of muscles associated with long-standing disuse. Following this she was prepared to involve herself in a programme of postural exercises, despite the fact that these initially caused her considerable pain. As important as the attitude to symptoms is *the attitude to treatment*. Behavioural treatment requires both effort and application from the patient. Neither of these is likely if the treatment that is being offered seems pointless, or if there is a pre-existing bias against this approach. An antagonistic attitude in the first assessment session does not mean that a behavioural treatment has to be rejected out of hand. However, it does mean that the first therapeutic task to be undertaken is that of engaging the patient in treatment and increasing motivation for the tasks ahead. A third area of enquiry should cover those *strategies that the patient already uses to cope* with symptoms. A young man with Gilles de la Tourette syndrome had learned to play the guitar. He noticed that if he played this and sung to himself sub-vocally his symptoms disappeared. This observation was of great value in helping him overcome his social anxiety and isolation which were an important part of the clinical picture. He was advised to arrive at a party strumming his guitar!

Primary focus on the symptom itself and the factors surrounding it does not mean that other factors in the past and present life of the patient are ignored by the behaviour therapist. Co-existing psychological problems, in particular depression, need to be taken into account, as does dependence on drugs or alcohol. The patient's underlying personality as well as key relationships may bear on the problem, as may significant life events and the social and cultural background. However, in contrast to psychoanalytic psychotherapists, the behaviour therapist is not seeking to impart some psychological meaning to the symptom, thereby promoting change through insight. Indeed whether or not the symptom has a demonstrable physical basis is, in a sense, irrelevant, provided that physical remedies have been shown to be ineffective or inappropriate. While not denying that a symptom may sometimes play an important part in the dynamics of a patient's life, the behaviourist is concerned with this aspect only insofar as it may influence active attempts to reduce distress or handicap caused by the symptom.

At the end of an assessment session the therapist will attempt to set up a *treatment contract*. Possible treatment approaches will be dicussed as clearly and openly as possible. The patient may well be provided with a booklet, describing relevant aspects of the anatomy, physiology, and pathology, of the condition from which he suffers. The booklet will also discuss psychological aspects of the problem, and outline alternative treatment approaches. An estimate of the number of treatment sessions involved will be given and the patient will be asked to involve other family members, if this seems to be necessary. In order to clarify the difficulties and to assist in monitoring progress, target problems will be agreed which can then be rated on a session by session basis as therapy proceeds. Finally, a diary will be designed (table I) to be completed on a daily basis before the next session.

Behavioural Techniques in Neurological Illness

Following the expansion in the number of behavioural techniques, and the broadening of the behavioural focus of interest to include internal cognitive phenomenon as well as external motor behaviour, there may be uncertainty and debate about whether a particular method is 'truly behavioural'. In practice, the style is a distinct one and can be discriminated without difficulty from psychotherapy based on the psychoanalytic model [*Sloane* et al., 1975]. In addition to *symptom orientation* which has already been discussed, there are a number of characteristic criteria. In the first place the treatment usually is *short term*. A typical course of treatment takes between 6 and 12 h, often given in weekly sessions of 1 h, though both the length and the frequency of sessions can be varied. Useful results may be obtained in a shorter time. For example, *Azrin and Nunn* [1980] report an improvement of over 90% in a group of patients with tics given only one or two 2½-hour sessions. Occasionally, particularly when new techniques are being tried out with difficult problems, treatment time may be much longer as in the treatment of brain defect states or reflex epilepsy when more than 50 h may be involved. Secondly, the therapy is *active, directive and structured*. The therapist gives advice, encouragement and sets tasks to be done between sessions as 'home-work'. In addition to talking, the therapy involves a variety of other activities including *relaxation, exercises, biofeedback procedures and role play*. Once goals and methods of treatment have been agreed therapy usually follows a predetermined plan, though the details may have to be modified if difficulties emerge. Although the therapist acts as director or coordinator of the treatment, other people, either professional staff or family members, may carry out an essential part of the programme, as in the involvement of ward staff in operant based treatment of pain [*Fordyce,* 1982]. Towards the end of a programme of treatment the therapist becomes less obtrusive, leaving the patient to take over increasingly the direction of treatment. Sessions are spaced at longer intervals, and after completion it is usual to follow-up at 3–6 months.

In any form of treatment it is important to try to distinguish specific from non-specific factors in treatment [*Gelder* et al., 1973], and behaviour therapy is no exception to this. Indeed, there is evidence that the behavioural style is a particularly effective means of establishing rapport [*Sloane* et al., 1975] and this is likely therefore to increase the non-specific or placebo effects of treatment. In addition, the assessment procedure, with its emphasis on clarifying targets, increasing understanding of symptoms, self-monitoring and heightening awareness of factors controlling symptoms, may have a significant though non-specific therapeutic effect. The power of non-specific factors is well shown in the treatment of migrainous and tension headaches using biofeedback (discussed in detail later).

Relaxation

A state of relaxation, characterised by measureable changes in a variety of physiological indices (pulse rate, GSR, blood pressure, and increase in alpha rhythm in the EEG) can be induced fairly easily in the majority of patients [*Heide and Borkovec*, 1984]. A number of methods are available. These may be either active or passive. Most behaviour therapists use exercises involving alternating muscle tension and release based on the progressive muscular relaxation technique [*Jacobson*, 1929]. Instructions used by the author are shown in table II. Passive methods involve the use of various types of imagery [*Kanfer and Goldstein*, 1980]. Judged by the end results, both subjective and physiological, the changes produced by both approaches appear to be equivalent. However, some individual patients who fail to respond to one method may respond to the other [*Heide and Borkovec*, 1984].

To be useful clinically it is important that relaxation can be self-induced. Having been taught the exercise in the clinic, the patient is asked to practice regularly at home. Audiotaped instructions are useful in encouraging this, particularly if the tape is made by the patient's own therapist. Having mastered the basic technique, the patient can learn to induce the state quickly using a cue word or signal such as taking a deep breath or saying the word 'relax'. This *cue-induced relaxation* can then be used in two different ways. Either the patient can be asked to imagine a threatening or anxiety-provoking situation, and then pair this with relaxation *(desensitisation)*. Alternatively, the relaxation response can be evoked in real life to head off an habitual tension-based response *(applied relaxation)*. Examples of both desensitisation and applied relaxation are found in the treatment of tension headaches and of chronic back pain.

Operant Conditioning

Operant techniques are derived from the experimental work on learning pioneered by *Skinner* [1938]. According to operant theorists, new behaviour is built up by selective reinforcement of desirable behaviour. Un-

Table II. Modified Jacobson's muscular relaxation – therapist guidelines

Stage 1	Preliminary discussion concerning the nature of anxiety and reasons why relaxation may be beneficial
Stage 2	Discussion of any apprehension or misconceptions concerning the relaxation process
Stage 3	General Instructions (a) 'This set of exercises is aimed to help you establish more control over your body' (b) 'The key element in these exercises is the process of letting go'
Stage 4	Specific instruction 'Make a fist with your right hand, tense it as much as you can, notice the feelings that this produces in the right hand which are likely to spread up to the right arm' 'Now in order to show you how you can control the amount of tension in your right arm I am going to ask you to let go the tension in the three stages as follows: one, let a little bit of the tension go; two, let a little more go; three, let the tension go completely and allow your arm to go floppy and relaxed' 'Now I want you to compare the sensations in the right hand and arm with sensations coming from the rest of your body'
Stage 5	The instructions given in stage 4 are now repeated for the left arm, right leg, left leg, abdomen, back, shoulders, neck, scalp, eyes, and jaw
Stage 6	The patient is asked to focus on sensations coming from their body at this stage and to notice any points of tension, and any parts of the body difficult to relax
Stage 7	If necessary, more attention can be paid to areas of tension by repeating the appropriate exercise or by devising a more narrowly focussed exercise to concentrate on particular pockets of discomfort
Stage 8	The use of fantasy can be employed at this stage to deepen the state of relaxation by asking the subject to imagine themselves in some situation where they would feel warm, safe and comfortable
Stage 9	The subject is asked to practice the exercises at least once a day if possible; a time of day should be chosen when the subject is neither too tired, nor likely to be disturbed for at least 20 min

wanted behaviour on the other hand should decline if it is ignored. In setting up an operant programme, for example in the treatment of chronic pain, the therapist aims to alter as much of the patient's environment as possible so that patterns of reinforcement are comprehensively altered. Illness-related behaviour, such as complaining, retiring to bed, or avoiding day-to-day tasks is ignored, while healthy behaviour is rewarded. Simple in concept, an operant programme needs care and thoroughness in organisation if it is to function effectively. Rewards need to be selected on an individual basis for whereas one patient may be influenced by praise, another may prefer something more tangible. Reinforcement may be negative as well as positive. Negative reinforcement is a confusing concept. It means the removal of something which would otherwise be unpleasant. A good example is that chronic pain could be negatively reinforcing for the patient in that it takes away the need to work. In therapy, negative reinforcement is used in the *time-out* procedure, in which the patient is allowed more and more time away from a boring environment as a reward for success in therapeutic tasks. Consistency in the application of reinforcers is also important and for this reason both clinical staff and relatives need to work together. The programme can be sabotaged unwittingly by an over-indulgent family or well-meaning but ill-informed nurse. Some operant programmes are based on token economies. In these, tokens act as a substitute for money and are used to reinforce a range of behaviours. such systems are versatile and flexible, and the amount of effort needed to gain reward can be adjusted to the individual patient and to the amount of progress that has been made.

Aversive Conditioning. In contrast to operant methods, aversive methods derive from the classical (respondent) conditioning studies of *Pavlov* [1928]. After enjoying a vogue some 25 years ago, aversive methods are rarely used by behaviourists at the present time. They have been abandoned because of ethical difficulties and because other more acceptable methods have been shown to be at least as good, if not more effective. Aversive methods are mentioned in this chapter because there are a number of case reports suggesting that they may be useful in the control of epilepsy. One of these cases [*Efron,* 1957] is worth examining in some detail since it illustrates both the difficulties with behavioural terminology and the importance of a detailed behavioural analysis. The patient, a 46-year-old woman with uncinate fits was able to identify a prodromal chain of events linked in a temporal order and culminating in a siezure. The events consisted of depersonalisation, forced thinking, olfactory hallucination, auditory hallucination and a head movement. She learned to interrupt this sequence by inhalation of a noxious odour and this reliably inhibited her convulsion. In fact, this therapeutic procedure differs from classical aversion therapy in two important respects. In classical conditioning the stimulus is given immediately before the response, whereas in this case it was given some time before. Furthermore, in this example the patient controlled her own aversive stimulus, rather than receiving an uncontrollable shock as did Pavlov's dogs. Thus, rather than being called 'conditioned inhibition', this procedure could more accurately be called *stimulus control.*

Habit Reversal. In contrast to the theoretical basis of both the methods described above, this technique is derived from clinical observation and simple mechanical principles. It appears to be highly effective in the treatment of tics [*Azrin and Nunn,* 1980]. In addition to the general behaviour therapy procedures which have been described, habit reversal involves a specific manœuvre for the immediate control of the unwanted symptom. The patient is taught to perform some action which is incompatible with the symptom. In the case of tics the competing reaction is the isometric contraction of muscle groups which are antagonistic to the tic movement. By practising in front of the therapist and then in front of a mirror, the patient learns to 'lock' the body in place so that not even a deliberate attempt to perform the tic produces any movement. Most patients quickly master this exercise and learn to achieve just the right amount of contraction, so that the tic is prevented but the controlling contraction is not apparent to an observer. The patient is then instructed to carry out this competing reaction for a period of about 3 min whenever the tic has occurred or is likely to occur. To be fully effective the patient has to learn to be sensitive to subtle cues which indicate that a tic is likely.

Massed (Negative) Practice. With this approach the unwanted movement is repeated over and over until the patient is tired. In the case of a tic or spasmodic torticollis, this would involve deliberate acting out the tic time and time again. Though lacking controlled evaluation, a number of case reports indicate that it may be of value. However, whether it operates through producing muscle fatigue or through increasing the patient's awareness of an abnormal movement is uncertain.

Assertion and Communication Skills Training

This approach has a strong educational flavour, and usually follows a programmed course [e.g. *Falloon* et al., 1977]. A start is made by describing the skills to be taught and their function in human relationships. A series of structured exercises are then carried out, increasing in complexity with the therapist using a combination of coaching, modelling and rehearsal, first in the clinic and later as 'home-work' exercises to be practised in the real world. Treatment is usually done in groups. Participants' achievements or difficulties are discussed systematically and success rewarded. The aim is not only to change behaviour but also to encourage observation of others in order to learn. Patients who lack assertion and communicate poorly, usually pay much more attention to their own thoughts and feelings, neglecting objective appraisals of the outside world. Subsequent sessions may be devoted to the recognition and handling of emotions and to the effects produced on others by taking different attitudes. Patients may be taught speaking and listening skills and be encouraged to recognise self-defeating attitudes. The training contains many elements of the cognitive approach (described below).

Cognitive Procedures. Cognitive methods of treatment derive from both theoretical and empirical sources. There is increasing evidence to show that not only do thoughts lead to changes in mood state but also that, in certain mood states, thoughts and memories associated with that state are much more frequent [*Beck,* 1980]. Arguments go on as to whether cognition or affect is primary. To the cognitive therapist, arguments concerning direction of causality are artificial in the sense that it is the circular nature of thought and mood which is postulated to be the key aspect of pathological anxiety or depression. The interaction could be tackled either by altering the underlying affective state or the thoughts. The latter are more easily accessible to psychological methods. In neurological conditions, the distressing thoughts associated with the primary symptom will be the therapeutic target.

An early example of the cognitive approach is to be found in the Rational Emotive Therapy evolved by *Ellis* [1962]. He focussed on the irrational way that his patients thought about their life styles, their ambitions and themselves. He demonstrated in a didactic or socratic manner the way in which anxiety, frustration and unhappiness derive from inappropriate attitudes or beliefs. Working on a short-term basis his style is essentially challenging and provocative. His influence has been based as much on personal charisma as on systematic evaluation of his method.

In contrast, the ideas developed in the Philadelphia School [*Beck,* 1980] have been tested in controlled studies with clinic populations, suffering from depression. *Beck* identified 'depressogenic schemata' which are mental constructs and concern the way in which the patients perceive their present personalities, their past and their future. In depressive states many of these perceptions are skewed or false. These perceptions are not challenged directly as they would be using the rational emotive method, rather the therapist sets the patient a number of tasks designed to demonstrate the invalidity of various beliefs. For example, the therapist may say 'It may be true as you claim that everything that you have done over the past year has been a complete waste of time but, let us sit down now and see what evidence there is to support that belief.' The patients are asked to carry out a number of homework tasks and to keep a diary of mood states. Inaccurate, self-defeating attitudes or thoughts which are associated with depression or anxiety are explored using Socratic questioning.

In addition to the ideas introduced by Ellis and Beck, other similar cognitive procedures can be used when appropriate. For example, *Meichenbaum* [1977], who has shown particular interest in the way that people cope with pain, stresses the importance of negative self-defeating thoughts. He encourages patients to modify their 'inner speech', asking them to practise self-statements even if at first they sound artificial. At the same time negative thought patterns are disrupted, using a range of 'thought stopping' strategies. Apart from modifying the frequency of different thoughts, these procedures help to enable the patient to distance themselves from their own thoughts by labelling certain cognitions as counterproductive. 'There I go again worrying about that pain and making myself anxious, let's try and see if I can think about something more productive.' Re-labelling of a different type can be important in helping to cope with the physical symptom such as anxiety and pain [*Suin and Richardson,* 1971]. Thus, 'the first sign of a heart attack' becomes 'a slight tension in my chest muscles' and an experience of panic can be re-labelled a feeling of 'excitement'.

Whereas traditional methods of anxiety management, both drug and behavioural, sought to abolish anxiety, the thrust of cognitive methods is to make symptoms controllable. As a means of achieving this the patient is first encouraged to re-think their understanding of the symptoms and then given something to do when the symptoms occur. It is quite possible these underlying processes are more important than the particular framework and strategy used in any one case.

Cognitive therapy means a general way of working with a fairly specific therapeutic focus. It also covers a number of techniques which overlap and are difficult to discriminate. When attempts have been made to evaluate cognitive methods in comparative studies, a combination of techniques is usually involved, since it is difficult and clinically inappropriate to tease out the individual strands that make up the therapeutic-package.

Biofeedback. Biofeedback methods are based on the postulate that if the subject is presented with high quality information concerning an aspect of physiological function then this function will be easier to bring under voluntary control. In the neurological clinic the three most important physiological variables are EEG, EMG and blood flow which are converted into visual or audible signals [*Johnston, 1978*]. Simple, non-invasive techniques of recording are usually used and training takes on average about 10×1 h sessions in a specially equipped laboratory [*Holmes and Burish, 1983*]. A number of commercially available systems are flexible, compact and portable and can be operated by the patient in their own homes. In its purest form, biofeedback involves giving the subject appropriate data and then reinforcing changes which occur in the desired direction, whether these occur randomly or as the result of some effort by the subject. It may be that increased awareness of, and attention to, a particular physiological process by itself provides a means of control. Very often, however, the subject is asked to try strategies such as a relaxation exercise or imagining that a certain part of the body is getting hotter and colder in order to produce a change. The biofeedback then simply shows whether or not this strategy has been successful. After enjoying a vogue in the last decade, interest in biofeedback is now declining as the result of disappointing performance in controlled clinical studies which are discussed below.

Evidence Concerning Effectiveness of Behavioural Methods in Neurological Conditions

Epilepsy

In attempting to assess the effectiveness of behavioural methods in epilepsy, one has to rely largely on case reports. A recent authoritative review [*Mostofsky and Balaschak, 1977*] described around 60 case reports but only 2 controlled group studies. Some of the case reports are themselves controlled using ABA or more sophisticated designs [*Hersen and Barlow, 1976*]. However, the majority are little more than anecdotal accounts with inadequate data particularly concerning baseline measures, medication regimens and exact diagnosis. Treatment methods often include a multiplicity of techniques and no attempt is made to control for placebo effects [*Mostofsky and Balaschak, 1977*]. Part of the difficulty lies in the nature of the condition itself. The epileptic patients that the behaviourists are asked to help form an extremely heterogenous group. They range from mentally handicapped institutionalised children to well-functioning adults. Seizures may be tonic clonic (grand mal), absence (petit mal), complex partial (psychomotor) or other type, and patients often suffer from a combination of different types. Fits may be with or without an organic basis; spontaneous or self-induced. Nearly all patients are on concurrent medication though there is only rarely any check to see if this is being taken regularly. In some patients it is easy to identify psychological factors in the genesis of fits, in others not. Finally, nearly all the patients referred for behavioural assessment are resistant cases that have failed to respond to other methods of treatment and represent, therefore, a hard core of 'problem patients'.

Faced with such heterogenicity, the conventional therapeutic trial in which patients are randomly allocated to one or other treatment groups or to a control is only of limited value. To give treatment methods a fair trial, individual treatment packages may have to be designed to suit a particular patient's problem as defined by the behavioural analysis. For this reason the well-designed controlled case report is of special importance in this field. A good example of how this can be done is given by a case reported by *Wells* et al. [1978]. They used an A-B-C-D design to study the effects of cue controlled relaxation on psychomotor seizures in a 22-year-old female who had suffered from seizures for 19 years. Behavioural analysis revealed that many fits were preceded by increasing levels of anxiety. Figure 1 shows both details of their design and the results. During the attention placebo phase (C) the behavioural technique was discontinued but the therapist continued to see the patient on a daily basis for 1 h to discuss general isues. Possible beneficial effects due to the therapeutic relationship by itself were further examined by substituting a male for a female therapist during phase (B'). Medication (carbamazepine 200 mg t.i.d.) was held constant throughout the experimental period. Independent observers confirm the patients self-reports of treatment gains, which were maintained over a 3-month follow-up period.

Techniques used in the treatment of epilepsy can be divided into three groups: operant, self-control and psychophysiological [*Pinkerton* et al., 1982].

Operant Methods. There are reports of the successful application of a wide range of techniques based on operant principles. All rely on a careful behavioural analysis. Attempts are made to modify the sequence of events leading up to the seizure or to modify the consequences. For example, in one of the earliest studies of treatment of this type [*Gardner,* 1967] the parents of a 10-year-old were trained to ignore seizures to which they had previously responded with great concern. Instead, they were encouraged

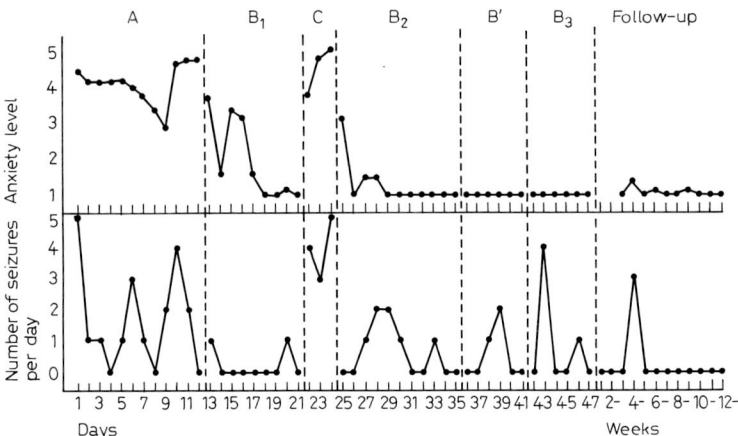

Fig. 1. Frequency of seizure activity and ratings of anxiety level across experimental phases: A=Baseline; B_1=cue-controlled relaxation; C=attention-placebo; B_2=cue-controlled relaxation; B'=cue-controlled relaxation with a novel therapist; B_3=controlled relaxation.

to pay more attention to desired behaviour. The treatment worked and when in a planned reversal the original pattern of response was restored, fits recurred within 24 h only to be eliminated by a return to active treatment. Some workers, particularly those treating handicapped children, have used aversive stimuli such as electric shocks or the more humane 'shake and startle' procedure, in which parents are taught to hold their child firmly by the shoulders, shaking them once vigorously and shouting 'no' [*Zlutnick* et al., 1975]. As in other operant strategies it is important to involve teachers as well as parents [*Balaschak*, 1976]. Punishment techniques have usually been used to interrupt the pre-fit chain of events, rather than to punish the seizure itself. However, programmes involving positive reinforcement or time-out procedures have been used successfully to reduce the frequency of seizures directly by rewarding fit-free periods. These are of value where it is not possible to identify or influence prodromal events.

Self-Control Methods. Anxiety management and cognitive procedures are the two techniques in this group. Relaxation is easily learned and may be particularly effective if used as part of a desensitisation programme

[*Parrino*, 1971] or in a cue-controlled style [*Wells* et al., 1978]. If thoughts centering around the consequences of the epilepsy, such as social stigmatisation, employment difficulties or low self-esteem, are causing anxiety and distress, then cognitive strategies may be of value. Cognitive procedures have only recently become popular, however, and their use in epilepsy is only mentioned in passing in the literature so far [*Pinkerton* et al., 1982].

Psychophysiological Methods. Instrumental feedback has allowed the development of a number of methods of treating epilepsy. One of the most promising and also one of the best researched concerns the effects of central cortical EEG feedback training. Neurophysiological studies in cats [*Wyrwicka and Sterman*, 1968], led to the conclusion that thalamic and cortical inhibitory elements are activated when the cats learn to increase the incidence of rhythmic 12–16 Hz sensorimotor rhythm (SMR) EEG activity. A number of reports indicate that this observation may have relevance for human epilepsy. Though the earlier of these reports was criticised because they failed to control for the placebo effect, an ingeniously designed study has met this difficulty [*Sterman and MacDonald*, 1978]. In this study 8 patients whose epilepsy had been poorly controlled with anticonvulsant medication for at least 3 years were included in a single-blind ABA programme. After 3 months baseline logging, they were trained to control different frequency bands by differential reinforcement using monetary rewards and other reinforcers. Three wave bands were used, 6–9, 12–15 and 18–23 Hz, and the patients were blind as to the bands used in their training. Results showed a significantly greater effect after training on the two higher frequency bands, after which there was a mean reduction in seizure rate of 75%. However, there was a marked individual variation in the response that was frequency dependent. Improvement was maintained at 3 months follow-up. SMR training is time consuming but patients can be given portable equipment to allow training at home.

The rare reflex epilepsies evoked by sensory stimuli may be improved by a conditioning treatment developed by *Forster* [1972]. If the precipitating stimuli can be precisely identified, a closely related stimulus is repeatedly presented until it loses its evocative quality. For example, a 21-year-old lady had a history of myoclonic seizures precipitated by biocular stroboscopic stimulation of frequencies between 15 and 35 flashes per second but was not affected by monocular stimulation at the same frequencies. Treatment involved extensive monocular stimulation both in the laboratory and at home where the television was set to 'roll' at the appropriate frequency. This training was followed by an improvement, which was, however, only temporary. In other cases, beneficial results have been reported with a variety of different stimuli, in which the intensity or the duration of the stimulus is gradually increased during training. This work involves complex apparatus and is time consuming (e.g. 60 h in a typical patient). It remains largely a research procedure awaiting controlled evaluation.

A simpler technique involves using biofeedback to convert paroxysmal activity to an auditory signal in patients in whom photically induced or spontaneously spike and waves could be recorded on EEG [*Korein* et al., 1971]. In this study only 3 out of 15 patients learned to control spike and wave activity and reduce seizures, indicating a rather limited place for this method. More promising results are reported in another study [*Cabral and Scott,* 1976] in which patients were treated with both relaxation and biofeedback designed to increase alpha rhythm and to hold alpha rhythm after anxiety-provoking stimuli. All 3 patients involved improved, and clinical imporvement was mirrored in their EEG records. However, it is not possible to say whether this improvement occurred from the relaxation, the biofeedback or from some non-specific effect.

In clinical practice therapists rarely restrict themselves to a 'pure' treatment approach consisting of a single technique. Results of a more 'naturalistic' approach combining operant, self control and physiological methods are reported by *Lavender* [1981]. 4 children at residential school, with a history of poor seizure control, were studied using an AB design. 2 of these children showed a significant reduction in fit frequency, which made their management on a day-to-day basis much easier. This study, in many ways, summarises the position regarding the behavioural treatment of epilepsy. Behavioural treatments can be said to be capable of making a contribution, though the extent of this contribution remains to be evaluated. A few patients may respond completely to behavioural methods, whereas others remain resistant. However, for many patients, if behavioural methods are included in general management, alongside conventional drug therapy, they may either reduce the need for anti-convulsant medication or improve the quality of the patient's life. It has been shown that no one behavioural method is the most powerful but that different methods are appropriate for different problems. Emphasis on the behavioural analysis of the problem may help both patients and their physicians to be more aware of factors of potential importance in the overall pathology of this distressing and disabling condition.

Tension Headaches

Recent psychophysiological findings in tension headaches have undermined the conceptual basis on which behavioural treatments have been founded [*Philips*, 1980]. These findings are timely in that they help to explain contradictions between different treatment studies. They also provide a firmer basis for research over the next decade. According to the traditional view [*Friedman*, 1962] sustained tonic muscular contraction was a necessary and distinguishing feature of tension headaches; the elevation of EMG recordings and the severity of the headache being closely associated. The evidence challenging this view is summarised in an excellent review [*Phillips*, 1980]. The main findings are as follows: (1) Patients diagnosed as suffering from migraine have higher muscular tension levels than patients with tension headaches. (2) At least 40% of tension headache patients have EMG levels indistinguishable from controls. (3) When tested in terms of response to imaginal stressors all headache sufferers show significant response, tension and migrainous alike. (4) When different aspects of the pain phenomenon are measured there is poor correlation between pain-related behaviour, for example medication rates, subjective complaints and physiological changes. These findings are those that would be predicted from a 'non-specific' view of pain [*Melzack*, 1973]. (5) The muscles of the head, neck and shoulders, thought to be involved in tension headaches, show a high degree of specificity in action. For example, frontalis and temporalis are uncorrelated at rest. Furthermore, key muscles elevated at rest, or when stimulated, coincide with the focus of pain in only 25% of cases studied.

These findings led *Philips* [1980] to suggest a possible theory which better fits the observations. According to this, some factor which she labels 'mental tension' is instrumental in producing both tension headaches and muscular responses. The latter occur only in those individuals with high muscular responsivity. Looking at tension headaches in this way shifts the previous preoccupation with muscular tension to wider issues and in particular to the nature and possible control of stressors.

Early case reports and uncontrolled clinical studies promised a great future for biofeedback methods in the treatment of tension headaches [*Sargent* et al., 1972]. Reports comparing biofeedback with no treatment on the whole appeared to confirm this promise, since 5 out of 7 well-designed studies showed that biofeedback was effective both in lowering EMG level and in improving headache symptoms [*Holmes and Bursh*, 1983]. However, these studies failed to allow for placebo effects and six further studies have shown that a credible placebo can have the same effect in reducing symptoms as frontalis EMG biofeedback. Typical of this group of studies is that reported by *Andrasik and Holroyd* [1980]. 29 patients were randomly allocated to three different biofeedback groups. The first were trained to decrease, and the second to increase, frontalis EMG. The third group were trained to decrease forearm flexor EMG. All groups were led to believe that they were being taught to decrease frontalis and each was effective in learning to control the muscle that was really involved. The headaches in all groups improved and there was no difference between feedback methods in therapeutic effect.

Further disappointment for the exponents of biofeedback has come from those studies in which its effects have been compared with relaxation. A meta-analytic review [*Blanchard* et al., 1980] concluded that there was no difference between the two treatments, despite the fact that in some studies biofeedback was more effective than relaxation in reducing tension in frontalis muscle. Adding the treatments together produces no extra benefit. In bringing about lower levels of headache frequency, duration and severity, relaxation alone was as effective as relaxation plus biofeedback [*Chesney and Shelton,* 1976].

It is premature to conclude from the above results that biofeedback has no part to play in the management of tension headaches. Relaxation needs no special equipment and is easy to teach. However, some patients who fail to respond to relaxation may respond to biofeedback [*Blanchard* et al., 1982]. Whether these patients are those with high muscular reactivity remains to be seen. In any case it is clear that patients with this diagnosis are not an homogenous group, although in the literature so far they have been treated as such. Another factor which needs to be taken into account is mood. While confirming the value of relaxation therapy, [*Jacob* et al., 1983] showed a less-favourable prognosis in those with associated depression.

No conclusions can be drawn about the mechanism of change, and the therapeutic factors responsible for it. A cynic could argue that the positive results are simply an example of the attention placebo effect, and that all that is needed is for the treatment to be credible to the patient. However, in a recent study in which a behavioural package of treatment was compared to self-monitoring alone and to traditional psychotherapy, only those patients who had received the behavioural treatment improved significantly [*Figuera,* 1982]. *It can be argued that patients benefit not only from learning how to control their headaches but also from learning more about the way they are precipitated and the effects the headaches have on their lives. Cognitive treatments may well be valuable in this regard.* In two separate comparative treatment studies, *Holroyd* and co-workers [1977, 1978] have shown that a cognitive package was more effective than either EMG biofeedback (despite its effectiveness in lowering frontal tension), a wait list control, or a group that was merely taught to monitor their headaches. Similarly, Smith and Denney [1983] show the value of careful analysis of stress factors in a case study reporting the successful treatment of traumatic headache. In this case, the factors involved concerned conflict with others at work; time pressure due to a demanding schedule, concern over a fiancee's outbursts of anger, and difficulties in relationships with mother and sister. Treatment consisted of relaxation together with assertive training which included modelling, role play, discussion and cognitive home-work tasks. Other workers have reported the use of relaxation-based techniques such as systematic desensitisation in controlling the stimulus leading to the headache, as well as in trying to modify the symptom directly. In the future it is likely that the efforts of behaviourists will continue in this direction.

Migraine Headaches

Much of the discussion concerning the behavioural treatment of tension headaches can be repeated as far as migrainous headaches are concerned. Biofeedback treatments which were enthusiastically introduced [*Sargent* et al., 1972] have been shown to be based on ill-founded assumptions and to be no more effective clinically than relaxation. Biofeedback methods in this case consisted of training finger temperature or temporal artery pulse control. Though these physiological variables can indeed be controlled through biofeedback, there is no evidence that this by itself is related to change in headaches. 'True feedback' training was no more effective than 'altered feedback' in reducing headaches [*Mullinex* et al., 1978]. In a double-blind study in which patients were taught either to increase or decrease skin temperature, both procedures produced an equal improvement in headache but no more than in a group who simply kept records but had no biofeedback [*Kewman and Roberts,* 1980]. This is hardly surprising since it has been shown that there is no relationship between finger temperature control and cerebral blood flow, as measured using a radioactive technique [*Largen* et al., 1978]. Learning to control blood pulse volume in the frontal branch of the temporal artery may be of more relevance and has been shown to have a slight advantage over EMG biofeedback of frontalis muscle [*Bild and Adams,* 1980]. Though better than wait-list controls, both relaxation and biofeedback cause similar improvement in migrainous headaches [*Blanchard* et al., 1978]. Here the beneficial effects must almost certainly be acting through improving the patient's general sense of well-being in a non-specific way, rather than through a direct action on the physiological events known to be involved in the production of migrainous symptoms themselves. Again, cognitive methods, particularly those designed to help cope with stress, may be of value [*Mitchell and White,* 1977], though their value awaits systematic evaluation. As for biofeedback, the authors of a recent review concluded that its use 'as anything more than a placebo treatment of migraine headaches does not seem justified at this time' [*Holmes and Burish,* 1983].

Chronic Back Pain

The behavioural perspective on chronic pain, elaborated particularly in treatment studies of low back pain [*Fordyce,* 1982] is as important as specific behavioural treatment techniques. Behaviourists distinguish four facets of the pain phenomenon. First is nociception which results from potentially tissue damaging energy impinging upon specialised nerve endings. Second is the experience of pain which is the perceived nociceptive input to the nervous system. Third is suffering, a negative emotional response generated by pain as well as other situations such as loss, stress and anxiety. Fourth is pain behaviour. This includes any overt behaviour related to the pain experience, and includes speech, facial expressions, posture, gait, taking medicines, seeking medical investigations and reassurance, refusing to work, avoiding exercise and retiring to bed. There is a good deal of evidence to suggest that these components vary independently [*Fordyce,* 1982]. Behaviour therapists attempt to modify the latter three, but not the first. They have used operant techniques, relaxation and biofeedback, cognitive methods and multimodal approaches.

An operant approach assumes that the frequency of pain behaviour is influenced by both positive reinforcement such as attention, medication and sympathy and by negative reinforcement which follows from the avoidance of work and responsibilities. Equally important is the fact that well behaviour has been extinguished through lack of encouragement [*Fordyce,* 1976]. Treatment programmes aim to alter contingencies in all three areas as comprehensively as possible. Several authors comment on the importance of involving the family [e.g. *Anderson* et al., 1977]. Most outcome studies report an improvement rate of around 70%

[*Follick* et al., 1983; *Anderson* et al., 1977]. Considering that most patients referred to these programmes are chronic and disabled sufferers who have failed to respond to other methods of treatment, these results look impressive. However, the best improvements are seen in activity levels and in reduction in medication. There is less decrease in the amount of subjective pain suffered and no patients reported less than 4 on a pain severity scale ranging from 0 to 10 (10 maximum) [*Linton,* 1982]. Not surprisingly, since it is difficult to avoid presenting the treatment in a punitive light, around 50% of patients either refuse to take part in such a programme or drop out before it is complete. Finally, of 10 outcome studies reviewed recently [*Linton,* 1982], 9 were methodologically weak, employing the one group pre- to post-test design. The only controlled study [*Cairns and Pasino,* 1977] compared two types of reinforcement; verbal encouragement and visual encouragement given by displaying progress on a graph above the patient's bed. The control condition consisted of a normal ward programme. Both forms of reinforcement added significantly to the normal ward programme, the verbal more than the visual. A combination of both types of reinforcement was more powerful still. It is interesting to note that two thirds of the patients had significant psychogenic factors in their problems, but that this variable did not affect outcome. Unfortunately, patient numbers were small and there was no follow-up. Thus, the present evidence indicates that operant methods by themselves may be useful in a minority of patients but further controlled work is needed to confirm this.

Patients involved in behavioural treatment programmes are those in which the pain had persisted for long past the expected healing time following acute trauma. In such patients it is likely that a pain-muscular tension cycle is playing an important part in the problem. If this is so, relaxation should be capable of assisting in treatment. Out of 10 studies in the literature reporting positive effects, 2 include a control. The first [*Nowen and Solinger,* 1979] showed back muscle biofeedback training to be significantly more effective both in reducing pain and muscle tension as measured by the EMG. However, these effects appeared to be independent, since at three month follow up the pain remained improved, while the muscle tension had returned to its pre-treatment level. The second study [*Linton and Melin,* 1983] examined the value of adding applied relaxation to regular ward treatment, comparing both with a wait list control group. The group of patients in the combined group learned to discriminate internal and external warning signals that indicated pain and to counter this with the relaxation response quickly and in a variety of different situations. This group reported a 28% reduction in pain compared to a 17% reduction in the group receiving ward treatment alone and a 23% increase on the wait list. Patients who had learned to relax also reported a change in the quality of pain in that although it did not go away altogether it was easier to tolerate. No studies have compared biofeedback with relaxation, although generalising from the literature on tension headaches it is likely that both methods would have similar effects. However, a recent case report [*Wolf* et al., 1982] illustrates a sophisticated use of biofeedback which may prove of value. Here EMG feedback was used to show abnormal patterns of para-spinal muscular activity during quiet standing and trunk movement, this then provided a basis for the correction of posture, which was followed by a reduction in pain.

Cognitive behavioural methods have only been investigated in a controlled way when used in combination with other techniques. In the best designed study, 36 patients were randomly assigned to three groups [*Turner*, 1982]. The first had relaxation treatment alone. The second had relaxation combined with a number of cognitive strategies including working towards individual goals, identifying cognitive and affective responses to pain and learning various ways of coping, such as the use of self statements or coping images. Both active groups were superior to a wait list group who completed ratings and were contacted by weekly telephone calls. However, only the cognitive behavioural group continued to improve in the follow-up period, when they showed double the amount of time at work and half the use of health care than they had before treatment.

As might be expected the worse the pain the poorer the prognosis. When 35 successes were compared to 35 failures, the factors negatively associated with outcome were duration of complaint, numbers of previous operations, level of base line self-report of pain, number of days lost per week from work, and dependence on drugs [*Maruta* et al., 1979]. In addition, high neuroticism in the spouse predicts failure [*Roberts and Reinhardt*, 1980]. The patient referred by a general practitioner after conservative medical investigation is a very different proposition to the multiple operated drug dependent patient with whom the behavioural therapist is often faced. Bearing this in mind, while behavioural approaches to back pain cannot be described as of proven value, they show considerable promise.

Tics

The literature concerning the behavioural treatment of tics is dominated by the work of *Azrin and Nunn* [1973, 1980]. In the first paper they describe the use of habit reversal in 12 patients with a variety of tics and habit disorders. These ranged from nail biting to head and shoulder jerking, in patients aged from 5 to 64 years. The technique produced quick and lasting improvement in all, 10 patients being symptom-free after only 3 weeks and the other 2 showing a 90% improvement. The authors contrast their results with those obtained using other treatment methods: psychoanalytic psychotherapy 25% after several months of therapy; aversion therapy 75%; and pharmacotherapy (usually with haloperidol) about 50%. As the authors recognise, their 'habit reversal' treatment package contains a number of additional specific therapeutic factors, including self-monitoring, increased awareness of the habit itself and the chain of events leading to its occurrence, and a detailed discussion of more general consequences of the symptom. In order to control these factors they conducted a second study in which 22 tic sufferers were recruited by a newspaper advertisement and randomly allocated either to habit reversal or to negative practice. All patients had the same general behaviour therapy procedures. The results were an impressive confirmation of the value of habit reversal (fig. 2). Others have reported similar improvement rates using habit reversal, in small groups of patients with tics [*Greenberg and Marks*, 1982], and in bruxism [*Rosenbaum and Ayllon*, 1981], so the technique is well established. One reservation, however, needs to be borne in mind. The patients treated by *Azrin and Nunn* were all suffering from miscellaneous tics. None of the patients suffered from blepharospasm, spasmodic torticollis or Gilles de la Tourette syndrome. Since these distinct disorders may have separate pathogenesis and be more refractory to treatment, it is not justifiable to compare *Azring and Nunn's* results with those of other workers who have tried to treat these distinct disorders.

For example, *Fielding and Gunary* [1981] reported the successful use of negative practice, combined with relaxation in 2 cases of blepharospasm. The author has used a similar treatment approach in 2 cases of spasmodic torticollis [unpublished]. On the other hand, in a 60-year-old patient with both blepharospasm and spasmodic torticollis, EMG feedback reduced the blepharospasm but had no effect on the torticollis [*Roxanas* et al., 1978], while, in contrast, another report describes the success of EMG feedback in 2 cases of hemifacial spasm, but its lack of effect in blepharospasm [*Brudny* et al., 1974].

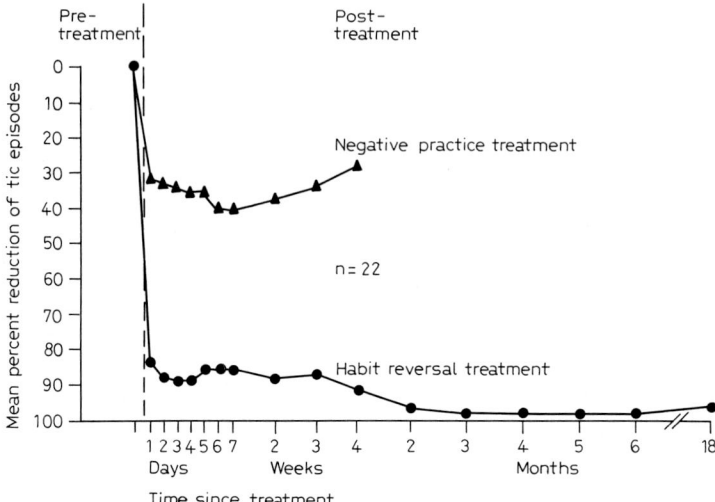

Fig. 2. Reduction of tics by two treatment methods. The tic frequency is expressed as the average percentage reduction relative to the pre-treatment frequency which is 0% reduction by definition. The vertical dotted line designates the time when treatment was given. Time since treatment is expressed in days for the first week, in weeks for the first month, and in months thereafter plus an 18-month follow-up. The day designated 'O' is when treatment was given. The upper curve is for the patients receiving negative practice and the lower curve is for those receiving habit reversal treatment.

Despite its dramatic and unmistakable clinical features, Gilles de la Tourette syndrome remains of uncertain aetiology. In such an obvious and distressing condition it is hardly surprising that emotional factors are involved [*Morphew and Sim,* 1969] though how much these are secondary and how much primary remains controversial. Behavioural treatments such as negative practice or habit reversal may focus on the symptoms themselves or may involve using relaxation, cognitive methods or assertive training to try to improve associated emotional problems. Case reports document both the success [*Clark,* 1966] and the failure of massed practice [*Feldman and Werry,* 1966] and, in 1 case, the effectiveness of operant methods [*Rosen and Wessner,* 1973]. These reports have to be seen in the light of the definite possibility of spontaneous remission and the apparent effectiveness of haloperidol [*Fernando,* 1976]. Despite the value of habit reversal in other tics, there is no report in the literature of its use in this syndrome. Although haloperidol may be remarkably effective in some patients, it is often poorly tolerated [*Fernando,* 1976]. It would seem, therefore, good clinical practice to either combine behavioural treatment with drugs so as to try to achieve positive results with the minimum possible dose, or to try a number of behavioural techniques on an empirical basis.

Straightforward cases involve the application of standard techniques in a routine manner. However, with more complex problems therapists need to be flexible and not only try out different methods but adapt existing ones. This is well illustrated in the treatment of a case of nocturnal bruxism [*Clarke* et al., 1981]. They showed that EMG-triggered waking was unhelpful by itself in reducing teeth grinding, but that if the patient was required to carry out an arousal task once awoken, then a maintained improvement in the bruxism was produced.

In summary, it can be stated that there is good evidence that habit reversal is the treatment of choice in simple tics. In more complex disorders of this type, behavioural methods are worth trying. Though not of proven effectiveness they are economical in terms of time and are free of side effects. They may be used either instead of or alongside of drug therapy, which incidentally is established on no stronger a scientific basis than behaviour therapy.

Writer's Cramp

Janet [1925], though not generally considered to be a behaviourist, was the first to describe the successful use of what would now be called a behavioural technique, in the treatment of writer's cramp. He suggested that after relaxation, the patient adopt a new writing posture. Then, in a systematic and structured way he gradually increased the patient's writing repertoire, starting with simple circles and progressing to normal script. Subsequently, a wide range of techniques have been described as effective, including relaxation [*Ajuriaguerra* et al., 1956]; avoidance conditioning [*Sylvester and Liversedge*, 1960]; systematic desensitisation [*Rognant and Ladouceur*, 1977]; EMG biofeedback [*Reaveley*, 1975; *Bindman and Tibbetts*, 1977]; habit reversal [*Greenberg and Marks*, 1982], and multimodal behavioural treatment [*Crisp and Modofsky*, 1965; *Cuttraux* et al., 1983]. Many of the patients who responded had received other treatment previously without help. However, all the reports are descriptive with no attempt at control.

Brain Damage

Interest in the psychological process by which learning takes place make the difficult challenge of retraining patients with psychological defects following brain damage a particularly strong one for behaviour therapists. Accepting the limits of both anatomical reorganisation and functional adaptation the aim of the therapist in this field will be amelioration rather than restitution [*Miller,* 1980]. A good deal of effort has been directed towards training in performing well on laboratory tests. Recently, researchers in the field have become aware that such tests may have little or no relevance to the patient's everyday life [*Powell,* 1984]. Learning to do well in a paired associate task may make no difference to the lack of ability to remember people's names.

Language and memory are the two functions which have attracted most interest. Faced with a dysphasic patient the therapist has three possible ways of helping. First is to reinforce and build up residual language function. This can be done by a systematic programme of instruction which can be combined with operant training. Though individual case studies report promising results, well designed controlled studies show no difference between active treatments and control procedures [*Sarno* et al., 1970; *Lincoln & Pickersgill,* 1984]. A second therapeutic possibility is to try to make use of the non-dominant hemisphere as in 'melodic intonation therapy' in which patients are taught to chant rather than talk. 8 patients with marked dysphasia following left hemisphere strokes, in whom spontaneous recovery was judged to have ceased, were treated in this way and 6 then showed further improvement [*Spark* et al., 1974]. The third strategy is to reject natural language altogether and try to construct an artificial one. Using a coloured paper system of symbols, 2 globally aphasic patients, neither of whom had any useful expressive capacity, were taught to make and use simple statements. However, the treatment did not have any effect on 5 other patients possibly because it was extremely time-consuming and the patients had to be discharged before the training was finished [*Glass* et al., 1973]. In an attempt to discover whether any intervention has therapeutic benefit, a large number of aphasic patients entering the neurological clinic in Milan were involved in a multimodal treatment programme or else received normal basic management. Unfortunately, the allocation of patients was on a geographical rather than a true random basis, and this may have accounted for the finding that although there were only small differences in psychological function between the groups the actively treated group did report greater improvement as far as practical, everyday, handicaps were concerned. The authors suggest that intervention may best be given early following brain damage but, in view of the fact that it is known that spontaneous recovery can continue for at least 9 months, this makes it vital for any further studies to evaluate this suggestion to be properly controlled [*Basso* et al., 1979].

In working with memory defects, two broad strategies are possible. The first is to enhance external techniques normally used as an aid to memory function [*Harris*, 1980]. Thus, patients are encouraged to use memos and diaries and to keep things in special places. The second is to use cognitive strategies. The use of visual imagery has long been known to enhance memory [*Patten*, 1972]. An example of the application of this, used in a multiple baseline design, is reported by *Wilson* [1981]. This patient had a severe memory deficit following removal of a left hemisphere tumour. Rehearsal alone was ineffective in learning names, but visual imagery enabled him to learn names of staff and friends. One, a Mr. *Pollard*, was taught by imagining a man on a bollard holding the letter P! A different cognitive technique, that of using structured enquiry, was used in a 22-year-old undergraduate who had a verbal memory defect following a road traffic acident. He was able to remember 94% of the main points of a prose passage after using structured enquiry, but only 36% after ordinary rote repetition.

Looking at this field as a whole, it has to be concluded that despite a great deal of effort we cannot claim that behavioural methods should be a standard part of a post-brain-damage rehabilitation programme. The methods are most likely to be rewarding in a small number of specially selected cases, for whom special techniques may be appropriate. A final example of this is the work of *Weinberg* et al. [1979] with a group of patients in whom right hemisphere lesions had led to visual neglect. Patients were trained on a reading task and a prominent marker such as a black line was used to stimulate further scanning. After practice the marker was gradually removed. Those treated did better than controls and, what is more, improvement generalised to some extent to other tasks normally impaired by neglect.

Conclusion

It is hoped that this chapter has shown that the status of behavioural psychotherapy in neurological disorders varies widely, from treatment of choice in the management of tics, to research interest only in the case of rehabilitation after brain damage. While some techniques such as aversive therapy and biofeedback have been shown to be largely redundant, others such as cognitive treatments are being developed and remain to be evaluated. The scope of the behavioural approach is wide. Not only may its methods be appropriate to problems such as anxiety which have an obvious psychological basis but, as in the treatment of epilepsy, they may be of value in problems which are organic in origin. It is striking, after reviewing the literature, to see how much behaviourists produce anecdotal case reports. This, despite their empirical tradition and strong criticism of those from a psychoanalytic tradition who base their ideas on similar sources. However, the development of the controlled case study makes it possible to draw more valid conclusions from case material. It also allows objective evaluation of treatment packages which are individually designed to cope with individual problems.

References

Adrasik, F.; Holroyd, K.A.: A test of specific and non-specific effects in the biofeedback treatment of tension headaches. J. consult. clin. Psychol. 48: 575–586 (1980).

Ajuriaguerra, J.; Garcia-Badaracco, J.; Trillat, E.; Soubiran, G.: Traitement de la crampe des écrivaines par rélaxation. Encéphale 45: 141–171 (1956).

Anderson, T.P.; Cole, T.M.; Gullickson, G.; Hudgens, A.; Roberts, A.H.: Behaviour modification of chronic pain. A treatment programme by a multidisciplinary team. Clin. Orthop. rel. Res. 129: 96–100 (1977).

Azrin, N.H.; Nunn, R.G.: Habit reversal. A method of eliminating nervous habits and tics. Behav. Res. Therapy 11: 619–628 (1973).

Azrin, N.H.; Nunn, R.G.: Habit reversal vs. negative practice. Treatment of nervous tics. Behav. ther. 11: 169–178 (1980).

Balaschak, B.A.: Teacher implemented behaviour modification in case of organically based epilepsy. J. consult. clin. Psychol. 44: 218–223 (1976).

Basso, A.; Capitani, E.; Vignolo, L.A.: Influence of rehabilitation on language skills in aphasic patients. A controlled study. Archs Neurol. 36: 190–196 (1979).

Beck, A.T.: Cognitive therapy of depression (Wiley, Chichester 1980).

Bild, R.; Adams, H.E.: Modification of migraine headaches by cephalic blood volume pulse and EMG biofeedback. J. consult. clin. Psychol. 48: 51–57 (1980).

Bindman, E.; Tibbetts, R.W.: Writer's cramp. A rational approach to treatment? Br. J. Psychiat. 131: 143–148 (1977).

Blanchard, E.B.; Andrasik, F.; Ahles, T.A.; Teders, S.J.; O'Keeffe, D.M.: Migraine and tension headache. A meta-analytic review. Behav. Ther. 11: 613–631 (1980).

Blanchard, E.B.; Theobald, D.E.; Williamson, D.A.; Brown, D.A.: Temperature biofeedback and relaxation training in the treatment of migraine headaches. A controlled evaluation. Archs gen. Psychiat. 35: 581–588 (1978).

Blanchard, E.B. et al.: Sequential comparisons of relaxation training and biofeedback in the treatment of three kinds of chronic headache, or the machines may be necessary some of the time. Behav. Res. Ther. 20: 469–481 (1982).

Block, A.R.; Kremer, E.F.; Gaylor, M.: Behavioural treatment of chronic pain. The spouse as a discriminative cue for pain behaviour. Pain 9: 243–252 (1980).

Brudny, J.; Korein, J.; Levidow, L.: Sensory feedback therapy as a modality of treatment in central nervous system disorders of voluntary movement. Neurology, Minneap. 24: 924 (1974).

Cabral, R.J.; Scott, D.F.: Effects of two desensitisation techniques: biofeedback and relaxation on intractable epilepsy follow-up. J. Neurol. Neurosurg. Psychiat. 39: 504–507 (1976).

Cairns, D.; Pasino, J.A.: Comparison of verbal reinforcement and feedback in the operant treatment of disability due to chronic low back pain. Behav. Ther. 8: 621–630 (1977).

Chesney, M.A.; Shelton, J.L.: A comparison of muscle relaxation and electromyogram biofeedback treatments for muscle contraction headache. J. behav. ther. exp. Psychiat. 7: 221–225 (1976).

Clark, D.F.: Behaviour therapy of Gilles de la Tourette's syndrome. Br. J. Psychiat. 112: 771–778 (1966).

Clark, G.T.; et al.: the treatment of nocturnal bruxism using contingent EMG feedback with an arousal task. Behav. Res. Ther. 19: 451–455 (1981).

Crisp, A.H.; Modofsky, H.: A psychosomatic study of writer's cramp. Br. J. Psychiat. 111: 841–858 (1965).

Cuttraux, J.A.; et al.: The treatment of writer's cramp with multimodal behaviour therapy and biofeedback. A study of 15 cases. Br. J. Psychiat. 142: 180–183 (1983).

Efron, R.: The conditioned inhibition of uncinate fits. Brain 80: 251–262 (1957).

Ellis, A.: Reason and emotion in psychotherapy (Lyle Short Press, New York 1962).

Falloon, I.R.H.; et al.: Social skills training of out-patient groups. A controlled study of rehearsal and homework. Br. J. Psychiat. 131: 599–609 (1977).

Feldman, R.G.; Paul, N.L.: Identity of emotional triggers in epilepsy. J. nerv. ment. Dis. 162: 345–353 (1976).

Feldman, R.B.; Werry, J.S.: An unsuccessful attempt to treat a tiquer by massed practice. Behav. Res. Therapy 4: 111–117 (1966).

Fernando, S.J.M.: Six cases of Gilles de la Tourette's syndrome. Br. J. Psychiat. 128: 436–441 (1976).

Fielding, R.; Gunary, R.: A behavioural treatment of blepharospasm. Two case reports. Behav. Psychother. 10: 184–188 (1981).

Figuera, L.: Group treatment of chronic tension headaches. A comparative treatment study. Behav. Mod. 6: 229–239 (1982).

Follick, M.J.; Zitter, R.E.; Ahern, D.K.: Failures in the operant treatment of chronic pain, in Foa, Emmelkamp, Failures in behaviour therapy, (chap. 17, pp. 311–334) (Wiley, New York 1983).

Fordyce, W.E.: Behavioural methods for chronic pain and illness (Mosby, St. Louis 1976).

Fordyce, W.E.: A behavioural perspective on chronic pain. Br. J. clin. Psychol. 21: 313–320 (1982).

Forster, F.M.: The classification and conditioning treatment of the reflex epilepsies. Int. J. Neurol. 9: 73–86 (1972).

Forster, F.M.; et al.: Clinical therapeutic conditioning in reading epilepsy. Neurology, Minneap. 19: 717–723 (1969).

Friedman, A.P.: Ad hoc committee on classification of headache. J. Am. med. Ass. 179: 717–718 (1962).

Gardner, J.E.: Behaviour therapy treatment approach to a psychogenic seizure case. J. consult. Psychol. *31:* 209–212 (1967).

Gelder, M.G.; Bancroft, J.H.; Gath, D.H.; Johnston, D.W.; Mathews, A.M.; Shaw, P.M.: Specific and non-specific factors in behaviour therapy. Br. J. Psychiat. *123:* 445–462 (1973).

Glass, A.V.; Gazzaniga, M.S.; Premack, D.: Artificial language training in global aphasics. Neuropsychologia *11:* 95–103 (1973).

Greenberg, D.; Marks, I.: Behavioural psychotherapy of uncommon referrals. Br. J. Psychiat. *141:* 148–153 (1982).

Harris, J.E.: Memory aides people use. Two interview studies. Memo. Cog. *8:* 31–38 (1980).

Heide, F.J.; Borkovec, T.D.: Relaxation-induced anxiety. Mechanisms and theoretical implications. Behav. Res. Therapy *22:* 1–12 (1984).

Hersen, M.; Barlow, D.H.: Single case experimental design. Strategies for studying behaviour change (Pergamon Press, New York 1976).

Holmes, D.S.; Burish, T.G.: Effectiveness of biofeedback for treating migraine and tension headaches. A review of the evidence. J. psychosom. Res. *27:* 515–532 (1983).

Holroyd, K.A.; Andrasik, F.: Coping and the self-control of chronic tension headache. J. consult. clin. Psychol. *46:* 1036–1045 (1978).

Holroyd, K.A.; Andrasik, F.; Westbrook, T.: Cognitive control of tension headaches. Cog. Ther. Res. *1:* 121–133 (1977).

Jacob, R.G.; Turner, S.M.; Szekely, B.C.; Eidelman, B.H.: Predicting outcome of relaxation therapy in headaches. The role of 'depression'. Behav. Ther. *14:* 457–465 (1983).

Jacobson, E.: Progressive relaxation (University of Chicago Press, Chicago 1929).

Janet, P.: Writer's cramp. Psychol. Healing *2:* 719 (1925).

Johnston, D.: Clinical applications of biofeedback. Br. J. Hos. med. *1978:* 561–566

Kanfer, F.H.; Goldstein, A.P.: Helping people change (Pergamon Press, Oxford 1980).

Kiewman, D.; Roberts, A.H.: Skin temperature biofeedback and migraine headaches. Biofeedback Self Regul. *5:* 327–345 (1980).

Korein, J.; Maccario, M.; Carmona, A.; Randt, C.T.; Miller, N.: Operant conditioning techniques in normal and abnormal EEG states. Neurology Minneap. *21:* 395 (1971).

Largen, J.W.; Mathew, R.J.; Dobbins, K.; Meyer, J.S.; Claghorn, J.L.: Skin temperature self-regulation and non-invasive regional cerebral blood flow. Headache *1978:* 203–210.

Lavender, A.: A behavioural approach to the treatment of epilepsy. Behav. ther. *9:* 231–243 (1981).

Lincoln, N.B.; Pickersgill, M.J.: The effectiveness of programmed instruction with operant training in the language rehabilitation of severely aphasic patients. Behav. Psychother. *12:* 237–248 (1984).

Linton, S.J.: A critical review of behavioural treatments for chronic benign pain other than headache. Br. J. clin. Psychol. *21:* 321–337 (1982).

Linton, S.J.; Melin, L.: Applied relaxation in the management of chronic pain. Behav. Psychother. *11:* 337–350 (1983).

Maruta, T.; Swanson, D.W.; Swenson, W.W.: Chronic pain. Which patients may a pain management programme help? Pain *7:* 321–329 (1979).

Meichenbaum, D.: Cognitive behaviour modification. An integrative approach (Plenum Press, New York 1977).

Melzack, R.: The puzzle of pain (Penguin, Harmondsworth 1973).

Miller, E.: Psychological intervention in the management and rehabilitation of neuropsychological impairments Behav. Res. Therapy 18: 527–535 (1980).

Mitchell, K.R.; White, R.G.: Behavioural self-management. An application to the problem of migraine headaches. Behav. Ther. 8: 213–221 (1977).

Morphew, J.A.; Sim, M.: Gilles de la Tourette's syndrome. A clinical and psychopathological study. Br. J. Psychiat. 42: 293–301 (1969).

Mostofsky, D.I.; Balaschak, B.A.: Psychobiological control of seizures. Psychol. Bull. 84: 723–750 (1977).

Mullinex, J.M.; Norton, B.J.; Hack, S.; Fishman, N.: Skin temperature biofeedback and migraine. Headache 17: 242–244 (1978).

Nowen, A.; Solinger, J.: The effectiveness of EMG biofeedback training in low back pain. Biofeedback Self Regul. 4: 103–111 (1979).

Parrino, J.J.: Reduction of seizures by desensitisation. J. behav. Ther. exp. Psychiat. 2: 215–218 (1971).

Patten, B.M.: The ancient art of memory. Archs Neurol. 26: 25–31 (1972).

Pavlov, I.P.: Lectures on conditioned reflexes (International Publishers, New York 1928).

Philips, C.: Recent developments in tension headache research. Implications for understanding and management of the disorder, in Rachman, Contributions to medical psychology, vol. 2, pp. 113–129 (Pergamon Press, Oxford 1980).

Pinkerton, S.; Hughes, H.; Weinrich, W.W.: Nervous system disorder, in Behavioural medical: clinical applications, pp. 215–232 (Wiley, New York 1982).

Powell, G.E.: Psychological assessment and treatment strategies in the rehabilitation of brain-damaged patients, in Rachman, contributions to medical psychology, vol. 3, pp. 173–191 (Pergamon Press, Oxford 1984).

Reaveley, W.: The use of biofeedback in the treatment of writer' cramp. J. behav. Ther. exp. Psychiat. 6: 335—338 (1975).

Roberts, A.H.; Reinhardt, L.: The behavioural management of chronic pain: long term follow-up comparison groups. Pain 1980: 151–162.

Rognant, J.; Ladouceur, R.: Traitement de la crampe de l'écrivain par désensibilisation. Perspect. psychiat. 5: 364–372 (1977).

Rosen, M.; Wessner, C.: A behavioural approach to Tourette's Syndrome. J. consult. clin. Psychol. 41: 308–312 (1973).

Rosenbaum, M.S.; Ayllon, T.: Treating bruxism with the habit-reversal technique. Behav. Res. Ther. 19: 87–96 (1981).

Roxanas, M.R.; Thomas, M.R.; Rapp, M.S.: Biofeedback treatment and blepharospasm with spasmodic torticollis. Can. med. Ass. J. 119: 48–49 (1978).

Sargent, J.D.; Green, E.E.; Walters, E.D.: The use of autogenic feedback training in a pilot study of migraine and tension headaches. Headache 12: 120–125 (1972).

Sarno, M.T.; Silberman, M.G.; Sands, F.S.: Speech therapy and language recovery in severe aphasia. J. Speech Hear. Res. 13: 607–623 (1970).

Skinner, B.F.: The behavior of organisms. An experimental analysis (Appleton-Century, New York 1938).

Sloane, R.B.; Staples, F.R.; Cristol. A.H.; Yorkston, N.J.; Whipple, K.. Psychotherapy vs. behavior therapy. (Harvard University Press, Cambridge 1975).

Smith, T.W.; Denney, D.R.: Relaxation training in the reduction of traumatic headaches. A case study. Behav. Psychother. 11: 109–115 (1983).

Spark, R.; Helm, N.; Albert, M.: Aphasia rehabilitation resulting from melodic intonation therapy. Cortox *10:* 303–313 (1974).
Sterman, M.B.; Macdonald, L.R.: Effects of central cortical EEG feedback training on the incidence of poorly controlled seizures. Epilepsia *19:* 207–222 (1978).
Suin, R.M.; Richardson, F.: Anxiety management training. A non-specific behaviour therapy programme for anxiety control. Behav. Ther. *2:* 498–510 (1971).
Sylvester, J.D.; Liversedge, L.A.: In Eysenck, A follow-up study of patients treated for writer's cramp by conditioning techniques in behaviour therapy and the neuroses, p. 334 (Pergamon Press, Oxford 1960).
Turner, J.A.: Comparison of group progressive-relaxation training and cognitive behavioural group therapy for chronic low back pain. J. consult. clin. Psychol. *50:* 757–765 (1982).
Weinberg, J.; Miller, L.; Gordon, W.A.; Gerstmann, L.J.; Lieberman, A.; Lakin, P.; Hodges, G.; Ezradii, O.: Visual scanning training effect on reading-related tasks in acquired right brain damage. Archs phys. Med. Rehabil. *58:* 479–486 (1979).
Wells, C.K.; Turner, S.M.; Bellack, A.S.; Hersen, M.: Effects of cue-controlled relaxation on psychosomator seizures. An experimental analysis. Behav. Res. Ther. *16:* 51–53 (1978).
Wilson, B.: Teaching a patient to remember names after removal of a left temporal lobe tumour. Behav. Psychother. *9:* 338–344 (1981).
Wolf, S.L.; Nacht, M.; Kelly, J.L.: EMG feedback training during dynamic movement for low back pain patients. Behav. Ther. *13:* 395–406 (1982).
Wyrwicka, W.; Sterman, M.B.: Instrumental conditioning of sensorimotor cortex EEG spindles in the waking cat. Physiol. Behav. *3:* 703–707 (1968).
Zlutnick, S.I.; Mayville, W.J.; Moffat, S.: Modification of seizure disorder. The interruption of behaviour chains. J. appl. behav. anal. *8:* 1–12 (1975).

Dr. John P. Cobb, BA, MRCPsych., Department of Psychiatry, St. George's Hospital, University of London, London SW17 ORE (UK)

Subject Index

Accident proneness
  characteristics 58
  definition 57
  head injury, association 61
    children 62
  inter-relationship, head injury/
    neurosis 59
  neurosis, association 60–64
  psychopathology 60
Adrenergic autoreceptors, locus coeruleus
  cell bodies 15, 16
Adverse life events, pathoplastic effect 53
Alcohol
  abuse, accident proneness 60
  head injury, reduced tolerance 63
  withdrawal, epileptic seizures 134
Alexithymia 54
γ-Aminobutyric acid
  antianxiety drugs, effects 5, 6
  extrapyramidal syndromes 123, 124
  Huntington's chorea 125
  seizure threshold, effects 147
Aneurysm
  depression, posterior communicating
    aneurysm 81
  psychogenic stress 78, 79
Anger, stroke, relationship 77
Angiography, emotional/personality
  factors 80–82
Antianxiety drugs
  action/mechanisms 3–6, 9
  clinical/biochemical effects 6
  hippocampal theta rhythm, effect 19
  see also Alcohol; Barbiturates;
    Benzodiazepines
Antidepressants, actions/mechanisms 12
Anxiety
  animal research, significance 2
  brain regions mediation, model 6–8,
    17–19
  cognitive therapy 163
  definition 4
  epilepsy, link 147
  hypertension, association 72
  management, epilepsy 166
  motor changes 121
  neural basis 5
  neural mechanisms 3
  noradrenaline, pathogenesis 125
  pathophysiology 121
  psychology 9
  psychotic interference effect 6
  septo-hippocampal system, role 6

Barbiturates
  antianxiety effects 3–6
  conditioned responses, effects 18, 19
  withdrawal, epileptic seizures 134
Basal ganglia, extrapyramidal disorders,
  role 121
Behavior
  changes, stimuli eliciting 3, 4, 7, 17

Subject Index

Behavior (cont.)
  conditioned/stress 17–19
  premorbid states, multiple
    sclerosis 86, 87
  systemic, controlling 1
  type A pattern 54
Behavioral inhibition system 3, 5, 7, 9, 88
Behavioral psychotherapy
  behavioral diary 153, 154
  cognitive factors 155
  methods 151
  rational emotive therapy 162
  symptom orientation, aspects 152
  techniques 157, 158
    aversive 160
    biofeedback 163, 164
    cognitive 162, 163
    massed (negative) practice 161
    operant conditioning 158, 159
    progressive muscular relaxation,
      therapist's guidelines 159
    reversing habits 161
    skills training 161, 162
  therapist's role 156
Benzodiazepines
  antiepileptic 147
  conditioned behavior, effects 18
  neuronal, CNS receptors, γ-aminobutyric
    acid, effect 5
Brain
  antianxiety behavior sites 6
  damage, behavioral therapy 177–179
  mechanisms mediating cancer
    resistance 21
  regions mediating anxiety, model 7–9,
    17–21
  see also Septo-hippocampal system

Cancer
  progression, psychological factors 20
  resistance, brain mechanism mediation 21
Carbamazepine, half-life/indications/
  serum levels 136
Cerebral arterial spasm, emotional stress,
  effects 78
Cerebrovascular accidents, *see* Stroke
Chronic back pain, behavioral therapy

  cognitive methods 174
  operant approach 172
  relaxation 173
Clobazam
  epilepsy, management 147
  half-life/indications/serum levels 136
Clonazepam
  epilepsy, management 147
  half-life/indications/serum levels
    136
Continuous reinforcement 17, 18
Coping
  definition 32
  denial/optimism 33
  problem focused 33

Delinquency, childhood, head injury
  history 62, 63
Depression
  after stroke 80, 81
  epilepsy link 145, 147
  helplessness, relevance 12–16
  incidence, idiopathic Parkinson's
    disease 114
  mechanisms mediating 12
  multiple sclerosis 86
  norepinephrine, role 125
  pathogenesis, serotonin 125
  reactive, head injury 63
  sleep disorders 146
  tyrosine hydroxylase, role 15, 20
  uncontrollable shock, model, DSM
    criteria 13–15
  Wilson's disease 116
Dopamine
  extrapyramidal syndromes 123, 124
  Huntington's chorea 118
  neurotransmitter, extrapyramidal/limbic
    systems 125
  tardive dyskinesia 119, 120

EEG
  cognitive stress 36, 37
  epilepsy, changes 34
  psychosocial factors, seizures 35
Epilepsy
  anticonvulsant therapy

Subject Index

principles 135–137
psychiatric sequelae 133
anxiety/depression 147
behavioral therapy 164
  operant 165
  psychophysiological 167
  biofeedback 168
  self-control 166
cognitive stress inducing 37
convulsions, causes 34, 134
definition 33, 133
depressive illness, link 145, 147
electroencephalography 142, 143
emotional triggers 35–37, 152
epileptoid character, concepts 140, 141
peri-ictal amnesia 35
personality changes 138
psychiatric disorders 138, 139
psychosomatic aspects 137, 144
seizures
  classification 134, 135
    generalized 135
    psychogenic 144
  electrophysiologic abnormalities 133
  psychobiology 139, 140
  stress associated 141–144
sleep deprivation, effects 36
Ethosuximide, half-life/indications/serum levels 136
Extrapyramidal disorders
  disturbed dopamine metabolism 124
  psychiatric disturbances 111, 112
  subcortical anatomical/neurochemical systems 121–126
Extrapyramidal system
  components/limbic system projections 122, 123
  neurotransmitters 123–125

Gilles de la Tourette syndrome
  behavioral therapy 176, 177
  choreic disorders/tics 111, 112
  coping 154–156
  dopaminergic dysfunction 118, 124
  obsessive-compulsive disorders 117
  underlying abnormalities 117, 118
Giving-up, given-up complex 53, 97, 98

Head injury
  accident proneness, association 61
  neurosis/premorbid personality 51
  psychological symptoms 63
Helplessness
  depression, relevance 12
  learned 61
  noradrenergic/non-noradrenergic transmission 13–16
  toughening up 13, 17
Hereditary chorea, see Huntington's disease
Hippocampal theta rhythm stress tolerance, role 19–22
Hippocampus, tyrosine hydroxylase activity 20
Huntington's disease
  γ-aminobutyric acid, role 125
  associated psychiatric disorders, 111, 112
    affective 115
    motor manifestations/pathology 117
    schizophrenia-like illness 115, 116
Hypertension
  emotional factors, association 82
  ischemic heart disease 73–75
  psychiatric morbidity, relationship 72
    depression 73
    environmental/occupational factors 74, 75
    hostility 73
    type A behavior 73, 74
  stroke risk factor 71, 74, 75
Hyperventilation, emotional arousal, epilepsy 37
Hypoglycemia, epilepsy trigger 37
Hysteria, organic disease, relationship 85

Idiopathic basal ganglia calcification
  associated psychiatric disorders 111, 112
    psychosis/dementia 116
  pathologic changes 116, 117
Idiopathic Parkinson's disease (IPD)
  associated psychiatric disorders 111, 112
    depression, incidence 114
    movement disorders, relationship 114, 115
  disturbed dopamine metabolism 124
  pathology 115

Subject Index

Intellectual assessment, head injury 50, 51
Interview Schedule for Events and
 Difficulties, essential features 30
Ischemic heart disease
 hypertension 73–75
 mortality/morbidity, role 76

Last straw phenomenon, disease
 relationship 54
Life change unit (LCU) scores 29
 life events, stressfulness 29
Life events
 adverse, pathoplastic effects 53
 definition 26
 difficulties, distinction 27
 health, relationship 27, 28
 multiple sclerosis, effects 42, 43
 social supports 31
 stressfulness, computation 28, 29
 theory, multiple sclerosis 91
Loss, experience, illness predictor 53

Mania
 cognitive/motoric manifestations 120
 noradrenergic/serotoninergic mechanisms 120, 121
 organic disease, relationship 85
Meige's syndrome
 associated psychiatric disorders 111–113, 119
 disturbed dopamine metabolism 124
 manifestations/pathology 119
Mental state, definition 2
Migraine headache, biofeedback, therapy 171, 172
Monoamine oxidase inhibitors
 action mechanism 12
 induced mania episodes 120
Mortality/morbidity, psychiatric symptoms 76
Movement disorders
 psychiatric disorders, association 111, 112, 120, 121
 see also Gilles de la Tourette syndrome; Huntington's disease; Idiopathic basal ganglia calcification; Idiopathic Parkinson's disease; Meige's syndrome;
  Postencephalitic Parkinson's disease;
  Progressive supranuclear palsy;
  Spinocerebellar degeneration; Wilson's disease
Multiple sclerosis
 associations/societies 102, 103
 emotional stress, role, 42, 87, 88
 environmental stress, effects 32, 41
 giving up response 97, 98
 inherited disposition 89
 life events, threat level 43
 Lorna-Doone syndrome 99
 onset/relapse, separation/engulfment threats 89–91, 106, 107
 life events theory, research 91, 92
 precipitant life event 93–96
 psychiatric disturbances 85, 92
  anxiety/depression 86
 psychological management 98, 99, 104, 105
  assessment 98, 99
  duration 103, 104
  form 100
  skills required 101
 psychosomatic factors 88, 89, 105, 106
 syndrome shift 88, 101
 traumatic life events 96, 97

Neocortex 5, 7
Neuropsychiatric illness, stress links 146
Neurosis
 accident proneness, association 72
 definition 54
 head injury, relationship
  alcohol/drug dependence 65, 66
  post-traumatic syndrome 63, 64
  somatic complaints 65
 hypertension, association 72
 mortality 55, 56
  physical conditions, links 56, 59
  psychosomatic explanation 53, 57
  suicide/accidents 56
 prevalence 54, 55
Nitrazepam, childhood epilepsy, management 147
Nonaneurysm intracranial bleeds, life stress, vulnerability 40

Subject Index

Noradrenaline
  brain levels, behavioral helplessness 15
  depression/anxiety, role 125
  extrapyramidal syndrome 123, 124
  hypothalamic 124, 125
  synthetase, behavioral stress tolerance 20
  toughening up effects, role 17
Noradrenergic tracts, origin 124

Obsessive-compulsive disorder
  Gilles de la Tourette syndrome 112, 117
  manifestations 121
  movement disorders 111
Organic brain damage 87, 88

Pain, behavioral changes, association 3, 4, 7
Paralysis agitans, see Idiopathic
  Parkinson's disease
Parkinsonian syndromes, movement
  disorders 111, 112
Partial punishment effect 17, 18
Partial reinforcement extinction,
  effect 17, 18
Personality factors, post-stroke
  depression, role 81
Phenobarbitone, half-life/indications/serum
  levels 136
Phenytoin, half-life/indications/serum
  levels 136
Phobias, symptoms, anxiety
  corresponding 9
Postconcussion syndrome 63, 64
Postencephalitic Parkinson's disease
  (PEPD)
  associated psychiatric disorders
    111, 112, 114
  disturbed dopamine metabolism 124
  etiology 113
  pathology 114
Post-traumatic neurosis 64, 65
Primidone, half-life/indications/
  serum levels 136
Progressive supranuclear palsy (PSP)
  associated psychiatric disorders 111, 112
  disturbed dopamine metabolism 124
  symptoms/pathology 118, 119
Pseudoneurasthenic syndrome 85

Psyche, definition 1
Psychiatric Epidemiology Research
  Interview (PERI), refinements 30
Psychiatric morbidity, subarachnoid
  hemorrhage 78
Psychosomatic disorders, multiple
  sclerosis 88, 89
Psychosomatic medicine
  definition 51
  history 52
  theories 53
Punishment, behavioral change,
  association 3, 4, 7

Reactive depression 63

Schedule of Recent Experiences
  (SRE) 28
  criticisms/flaws 29
Schizophrenia
  dopaminergic neurotransmitter
    systems mediating 120
  gait/posture changes 111, 112, 120
  organic disease, relationship 85
Septo-hippocampal system
  anxiety, role 6
  stress tolerance, role 18–22
Serotonin
  depression, pathogenetic role 125, 146
  extrapyramidal syndromes 123, 124
  synthesis 125
Shock
  emotional, multiple sclerosis 41
  uncontrollable, depression model 14, 15
Sleep deprivation, epileptogenicity
  36, 37, 146
Social environment
  health relationship 32, 33
    coping 32
  research subdivisions 26, 27
Social Readjustment Rating Questionaire
  (SRRQ) 28
Social Readjustment Rating Scale
  (SRRS) 28
Social supports 27
  health changes, relationship
    27, 31, 32

Sodium valproate, half-life/indications/
  serum levels 136
Somatic disease, association psychologic
  disturbances 1
Spinocerebellar degeneration, psychiatric
  disorders 111, 112, 118
Stress
  behavioral tolerance development 17–22
  body response 54
  cognitive, epileptogenicity 36, 37
  emotional
    multiple sclerosis 42, 43
    stroke, role 38, 78
  environmental
    health effects 28–31
    multiple sclerosis 41–43
  neuropsychiatric illness, links 146
Stroke
  behavioral/psychological contributions 41
  components 37
  consequences, affective changes 79, 80
  emotional factors 38, 75
    pressurized pattern 76
  genesis, life stress role 38
  hypertension predisposing 75
  life style factors 77
  personality factors, association 77
  risk factors 71
  survivors, depression/personality
    factors 81
Subarachnoid hemorrhage
  emotional stress/psychopathology 78
  severe emotional shock, role 39

Suicide
  Huntington's disease 115
  incidence, head injuries 62
Sulthiamine, half-life/indications/
  serum levels 136
Syndrome shift 88, 101

Tardive dyskinesia
  disturbed dopamine metabolism 124
  etiology/neuropathology 119
  manic-depressive illness 111, 112, 119
  stress/depression, effects 120
Tension headaches
  behavioral psychotherapy
    biofeedback 169–171
    relaxation 174
  symptoms diary 152, 153
Tics, habit reversal, results 175–177
Toughening up, stress tolerance
  13, 17, 20
Tricyclic antidepressants, induced
  manic episodes 120
Type A behavior
  frequency, post-stroke 77
  ischemic heart disease 73
Tyrosine hydroxylase, role,
  depression 15, 20

Wilson's disease, associated
  psychiatric disorders 111, 112
  depression/mania 116
  pathologic changes 116
Writer's cramp, behavior therapy 177